eat well
stay young

eat well
stay young

michel | **montignac**

Montignac Publishing (UK) Ltd

First published in 2001 by
Montignac Publishing (UK) Ltd
2 Mill Street London W1R 9TE

First Published in France under the title:
"Mangez bien et restez jeune"
1996

Text © Nutrimont/Montignac Publishing UK Ltd
Translated by Stuart Rothey

Design by Design Principals, Warminster

ISBN 2-912-737-05-2
EAN 97829 12737052

www.montignac-publishing.com
info@montignac-publishing.com

Contents

Introduction

Jeanne Calment has just celebrated her 125th birthday. It is a celebration in which we all share as fellow human beings. However, the lady also happens to be French and that must be cause for a certain amount of national pride in France.

To recall her nationality, however, would be of little significance were it not for the fact that statistics show that the inhabitants of France are less unhealthy than those of other industrial countries. This piece of information would scarcely warrant mention, were we not to add that this official *doyenne* of the human race has always lived in Provence, in the south of France, an area which has long been an arch exponent of the healthiest way of eating in the world - namely, the Mediterranean diet.

As many of us now join the vast club for fifty-year-olds, it is reassuring to know that the great-grandparents of some of us are still alive. This helps reinforce the feeling that we are still young. Furthermore, since the ranks of the patriarchs are visibly growing all the time, it no longer seems so unreasonable that we too may all reach the hundred mark one day. However, if we are all agreed we should live that long, then our aspiration must implicitly be conditional on our being in good health. The idea of merely surviving is quite unacceptable.

It is as well to remember, however, that in our age there are signs that should give cause for concern. For although we are able to prolong life beyond what was imagined possible at the beginning of the twentieth century, paradoxically our species has never been so ill. The statistics are equally disquieting: certain illnesses which formerly appeared late in life now appear earlier and earlier. This phenomenon is particularly pronounced in a country like the United States, where over the age of sixty - and sometimes before that - the population is in a state of decrepitude that is particularly worrying.

However, if the problem has been clearly identified, an effective solution has yet to be found. Though the medical and pharmaceutical industries have never been so active, inventive and productive, all is in vain. Health expenditure continues to be an ever-increasing burden.

The pathologies are known for the most part. Screenings have been mastered and therapies have been developed. Phenomenal progress has been made in surgical techniques, as well as in treatments, care and medications. But at the end of the day, the problem still remains unresolved: we know how to prolong life, but we are unable to ensure a good standard of health.

And yet the solution is always there and has never left us. It is modern man who in his scientific arrogance has deliberately disdained and ignored it. It is a matter of good sense and reason; one might even say wisdom.

The solution is quite simply on our plate, because it lies in what we eat - in the quality of our food. As Hippocrates said five centuries before Jesus Christ, "food is our best medicine".

We have reason to be proud of our doctors, of our researchers and of all our scientists who, by dint of their courage and determination over the course of half a century, have caused scientific knowledge to progress by leaps and bounds. They have pushed back the boundaries of medical knowledge in a quite exceptional manner, but at the same time they have obscured what is of fundamental importance: the food factor. They have forgotten one of the basic premises of existence for a living organism, whether animal or vegetable; namely, that its survival and health are closely linked to the quality of its nourishment.

Since the end of the last world war, food production has undergone a complete revolution. Two causes lie at its roots: one is the sharp increase in the population in the West - the so-called "baby-boom", which has caused public bodies to encourage mass-production; the other is the phenomenal increase in urbanisation within the space of a few decades, which has emptied rural areas and filled the cities, creating a significant imbalance between the areas of production and the areas of consumption.

In order to produce more, we have mechanised to excess, fertilised with chemicals, engaged in chemical warfare with our environment using excessive amounts of pesticides, insecticides and weed-killers. In addition, we have selected seeds through controlled hybridisation, with the sole aim of increasing yields.

In order to conserve foodstuffs whilst transporting them from the areas of production to the areas of consumption, we have introduced harvesting before crops have matured, artificial ripening, refrigeration, freezing and a whole range of different industrial practices such as ionisation. These are used to give an artificial impression of freshness to products that in normal circumstances would have rotted.

At the end of the chain, the food industry has not been idle either. It has introduced new ways of conditioning and conserving food by using additives to improve appearance, enhance taste artificially or, again, prevent food decomposing naturally.

At the same time, animal production has become intensive, creating confined areas in which to raise animals and introducing hormones and antibiotics to help increase production.

The result of this technical revolution is undoubtedly progress. It must be recognised that in effect nobody in the Western world suffers hunger - not even those who have the misfortune of being without work and perhaps no permanent home. The superabundance of food that characterises our affluent society is sufficient to feed everybody, even those who do not have the means.

However, the other side of the coin is that, although we may be certain of having the quantity, every day that passes we become more aware that we lack the quality. The nutritional quality of foodstuffs is in fact so low that we might even consider we have already reached danger level. This means the food offered to us today no longer caters for the nutritional needs of our bodies. Apart from the energy that allows us to survive, our bodies are deprived of the vital elements essential to keep us in good health.

On the other hand, it would be an exaggeration to consider all foods available to us as suspect. Those foods that deserve mention because of their poor nutritional content are essentially those that have been subjected to intensive production methods and more often, those that have been modified or transformed by industrial methods. The others that fortunately still exist are not only acceptable but even recommended.

Eating habits have changed considerably during the course of fifty years. However, what is unfortunate is that people these days are more inclined to choose bad foods instead of good. And yet, in all the cases where people have been sufficiently convinced to take positive steps to improve their diet, the results obtained have been sufficiently encouraging to warrant continued implementation of the changes.

During the first part of life, usually before we reach our fifties, the body copes with the deficiencies and inadequacies of a poor diet without giving undue sign of any problems. It compensates in part for these deficits by drawing on its reserves, which explains why so few signs are detectable before rapid deterioration sets in.

And then, one day, the flashing lights are switched on - though the situation is really not taken seriously until there is a major alert. This is the time for bad surprises, for disappointments and for regrets. It can also be a time for belated resolutions, since it is never too late to start making good decisions. However, whatever the scenario, it would have been far better had we not been obliged to make these decisions with our backs to the wall.

This book has been written to help prevent that situation ever arising.

And then there are a good number of you who, much to your surprise, have passed the fifty mark and are still in the prime of life - still in complete possession of all your physical and mental faculties.

This book is also written for you, to help you take stock of the situation, to realise that after half a century of good and loyal service from that fantastic machine you call your body, it would be wise to offer it at least a programme of preventative measures, even if you are unable to give it the proper check-up and complete service it deserves. Your body has a logic that reason should understand.

However, this book is also addressed to those who are a little more advanced into the second half of their life, and particularly those who have a few niggling worries about their health. For them, the advice contained in this book may not lead to a complete recovery, but it will at least afford them a degree of remission.

In any event, all will discover that the food factor is of paramount importance with regard to health and that some changes in this area of their lives will be sufficient in order to approach life full of optimism once more. Quite painlessly, they will come to realise that the only way of staying young and in good health is simply to eat well.

PART ONE
The Roaring Fifties

The baby-boom generation is in the process of passing the fifty-year-old mark. The majority feel themselves to be eternally young: their idols of yesterday are still those of today; they themselves do not appear to change, or only very little.

After having blown out the many candles on the big cake and as soon as the last strains of "Happy Birthday" have died away, the recipient of all these good wishes undergoes the ritual question: "What does it feel like to be fifty?". And as in previous years, the ritual answer comes back, laced with smiles: "It feels just the same! It feels as if I were still twenty!"

It is true, yet false. For when we, the birthday candidates, come face-to-face with ourselves, we cannot help but wonder. The smallest weakness in our body causes doubts to stir within the soul, dragging with them on the odd occasion a certain anguish. For it is during this period in our life that we are torn between the received ideas of a culture that views age without pity on the one hand and our profound feeling of well-being and hope on the other.

It is a critical age; you are neither one thing nor the other - neither young nor old. The body has acquired a few wrinkles, the hair is greying if not yet white, and glasses have become unavoidable crutches. Is it perhaps the time to quieten down, to prepare a retreat and look forward to a well-earned rest...and eternity?

Nothing could be more wrong! At fifty, your drive is not declining - quite the opposite! This is not the time to fade away: it is the time for development. It is not in fact a critical age but a decisive age.

There are two periods of youth in life. The first one, known to everybody, and the second one, less well known, which starts at fifty.

First youth is a hard, merciless age. It is the time for tilling the soil and sowing the seed. It is a time for experiences, discoveries and apprenticeships. It is a time when we are prisoners of our surroundings, our family, our masters, institutions and systems. We are also prisoners of ourselves, of our instincts or, at very least, our impulses.

Second youth is, on the contrary, the age of harvests. It is the period in which the individual comes to fullness and maturity. It is a time of transformation. Knowledge, experience and awareness bring pleasure. The individual is free. For although we may always belong to a group, we are no longer dependent. We are also free in our minds and our relative vision of things gives us the detachment necessary for objective decision-making. The mastery of our ideas, of our tastes as of our nature, helps us to control ourselves better. Knowing how to manage our desires and passions give reason a greater chance to influence our lives.

The fifties is an age of dynamic wisdom, when considered decisions are made in the light of knowledge and experience, unaffected by external obligations. Men and women of this age are endowed with all the powers and all the virtues. Far too many among their generation consider themselves half-old already and even begin to entertain an inferiority complex.

However, they must release themselves from this burden and discover - as Georges Barbarin used to say - that in fact "life begins at fifty!". But as with everything in this life, the happiness of second youth does not come entirely of its own accord. It must be allowed to express itself and to grow. And to come by it, there are three elementary rules to be followed that for sake of convenience, we will promote into principals.

TURN YOUR BACK ON THE PAST

The biggest danger to guard against on becoming fifty is to remain a prisoner of the past. The memory of the first fifty years can too often constitute the constant reference of our thoughts, the life belt that we grasp and that then prevents all further progress.

How can you enjoy the present and prepare for the future if you stay a prisoner to your past? After all, the best way to have a car accident is to drive looking only in the driving mirror. The past is relevant only insofar as it has a bearing on the present. It is the apprenticeship, the knowledge and the experience acquired in the past that, once synthesised in the subconscious, can be drawn upon by the spirit when required.

What is reprehensible is not so much the past in itself, which is necessary for the lessons it brings, but the continual harking back to old memories which help to inspire and cultivate that worst of all enemies - nostalgia. The past is, in fact, a deception and its memories a snare, for the image it gives of what has been lived is false, deformed, idealised and embellished.

How can you advance and make the necessary objective choices to manage the present and prepare for the future, if you constantly refer to a sugary past purged of all the realities of existence, which does not give us things, people and events but rather a subdued rosy vision of life? Some even have a psychopathic approach to their past, where reality is not only deformed, it is reconstructed to the point that they invent stories which through repetition they end up believing themselves. Generally these are people who are uncomfortable with their persona and whose lack of self-esteem pushes them to invent a glorious past for themselves or their family. If they entertain this false past, convincing themselves of its reality, it is often to compensate for the mediocrity of their present existence and their inability to confront the future.

They are the same people who travel only in order to take photographs and then show them to their friends, inventing the pleasure which should have accompanied the event but which they have never had, for they only really live in a nostalgia for what never existed. In order to escape the harsh realities of life which they have never been able to accept, they are the people who invent a golden youth with parents who were an ideal couple, when in fact they never ceased arguing, fighting and living from hand to mouth.

In these conditions, how can you confront the second part of your life with courage, realism and objectivity, if you have spent the first part lost in dreams, illusions and self-deception? For some of them, a visit to the psychoanalyst should be compulsory. This is why it is necessary not only to doubt the past but above all, to question all feelings of nostalgia for they systematically pull us backwards just when we should make a big step into the future. The present and the future are the only moments in life that deserved to be lived.

Look at the door that is opening and ignore forever the one that is closing.

REFUSE TO ADOPT MIDDLE-CLASS ATTITUDES OR TO BE CONVENTIONAL

The baby-boom generation will figure in history as a privileged generation on the economic front. Those fifty-year-olds who have not succeeded in making a place for themselves in the sun or at least protect themselves financially are a rare species. There are certainly many who have been sacked, but their trial has usually been more a moral and social one than a financial one.

Twenty-five years ago it was enough to want to work in order to find employment, and to invest a modicum of effort in order to succeed. With a few years of experience, the workman became craftsman, manager and owner. All types of work gave us the opportunity of making money and getting out while the going was good.

However, the consequence of this rise in the standard of life in France, with its matching job-protection scheme known as the *protection sociale*, was a massive increase in the number of people with middle-class aspirations. Having burst upon the world, this phenomenon appears already to be collapsing in on itself, on its preconceived ideas, laws and privileges.

From acquiring property to dabbling as a minor player in stock and shares, and then entering into savings plans and life assurance policies, certain pot-bellied fifty-year-olds have fallen into step with that group of people of independent means who flourished in the last century, by actively cultivating security and immobility. Little by little they have allowed themselves to be wrapped up in a straitjacket of ease and comfort, and seduced by the rhythm of school holidays, pleasures and above all by the interminable evenings spent in front of the television with their slippers on. It is a France that purrs with pleasure and sleeps contentedly, which caricaturists lay bare from time to time.

Staying young is above all a refusal to adopt middle-class attitudes. However, this calling into question must be preceded by taking stock, by analysing the situation as objectively as possible and by confronting the real issues. When you reach the age of fifty, whether you are a man or a woman, it is still possible for you to start your life again for it is never too late to do things better. It is just a question of having the will. In any case, those who have done it have had no regrets and have shown that the chances of success are high because at this time of life, choice will benefit from mature judgement.

Professionally it is the best moment to launch out and realise the dream of your life: to become independent. In any event, the question will have to be examined seriously should an accident along the way result in you losing your job.

As far as couples are concerned, the choices should also be examined with objectivity and realism. If the union has been constructed on fragile foundations where misunderstandings and incompatibilities persist, leading in their turn to frustrations, sourness and resentments, then there is still time to be brave and recognise failure. Think of the future. Look around at the sad couples that end their lives loathing one another and spending their time engaged in mutual destruction. On the other hand, if the union enjoys solid foundations, then take stock of the situation, repair where necessary and cherish what is good.

One of the important decisions that can also be part of the renaissance is moving home - not forced by events but chosen deliberately as your lifestyle has matured and your quality of life has improved. Why not realise that dream (shared by all the family) which consists of going to live in a big house in the country? Why wait to retire before taking such a step? All those who have had the experience would not go back for all the gold in the world and it is surprising how many of their friends envy them or follow in their footsteps.

On the other hand, in order to stay young it is also important that we refuse to conform. We should call into question all the rules that govern our social life, retaining only those that appear really necessary - in particular, those that involve consideration and a respect for others. However, let us dispense with all ridiculous obligations, social gymnastics and futile conventions.

At the age of twenty-five, we are still trying to find ourselves. That is why we need to show we belong to a system or group, which will require respect for all the conventions if we want integrate better. But when we reach the age of fifty, we should be able to rise above outdated principles and traditions, received ideas and social conventions.

After all, it should be possible to decide to be ourselves and still remain civilised.

TAKE CARE OF YOURSELF

We have to look no further than the Judaeo-Christian culture, which has been a fundamental part of Western life over the last two millennia, to explain the difficulty that many of our contemporaries still have in looking after their bodies. For many centuries, only the spirit was considered worthy of interest. The human body was regarded as being just a vile accessory with degrading functions shared with the animals. It was therefore better ignored.

For a long time, only ladies of questionable virtue could allow themselves to violate this austere existential programme, by using deceits designed to underline their charms. Since they were engaged in selling their bodies, it was understandable that they should highlight the value of the merchandise on offer.

Fortunately modern attitudes have evolved during the course of recent decades, so that interest in one's appearance has become quite acceptable even if the Church may regard it a sin of pride. Even a certain tolerance is admissible in the case of men, who can now use toiletries without derision.

All those who decide to take a course of yoga or relaxation therapy are amazed that the first lessons are focused on the discovery of the body. Those that fail the apprenticeship phase of these relaxation techniques are always those that are unable to "integrate their body image", to admit that their body and their spirit are one and proceed to reintegrate one within the other to make a whole.

The two bodies - spiritual and physical - are in effect inseparable for when one receives a stimulus, the other may well reveal the symptom.

Discovering our body, listening to what it has to say, accepting it and cherishing it, is part of an inescapable journey of finding harmony in ourselves. If individuals do not love themselves - or at least, do not admit it - it is a sign that their bodies have not been taken into account for some time. For how can body and soul love each other if they do not know one another and have ignored each other for so many years that they are now total strangers?

To remain young, it is necessary to act sometimes with regard to the body and sometimes with regard to the spirit. But for each step to be completely effective, an essential precondition is that body and spirit should be reunited. With a child, this unity exists naturally. It is education and above all culture that progressively disassociate the two. It is from then on we can understand that to be at ease with ourselves is primarily a question of being in harmony or joined within ourselves.

The malaise of adolescents is essentially a disharmony between a foreign body - an adult body that has appeared too quickly - and a spirit that has not been able to integrate with it, mainly because the spirit is still that of a child.

With an adult who is fifty years old, disharmony is more or less pronounced but can be accentuated by the physiological changes that occur at this time of life. The best way of remedying the situation will be to take stock first of all, and then work on a course of harmonising again, with the help of techniques such as yoga and relaxation therapy.

However, if we are concerned with our body, we are inevitably concerned with our health and, as a consequence, with the way we eat. Since Hippocrates said "we are what we eat", it is clear that our food, if it is good for our body, it will also be good for our spirit.

In France, those now in their fifties have had the good luck of being brought up in a specifically French dietary environment, whereas their children have grown up in a cosmopolitan environment with a strong North American character. This means that men and women of this earlier generation have preserved in their dietary habits the principles that were handed down by their parents and grandparents. For them, as for the majority of Frenchmen, a meal is not merely the satisfying of a primary physiological function as it is in the States, where a meal is merely seen as a way of satisfying hunger by eating any old food. For them it has not only a social and convivial dimension, it also has a hedonistic one, in the sense that it is a fascinating part of the quality of life. For them, it will be easy to add a further dimension to eating - to make food and the quality of food an essential factor in the maintenance of health.

As we shall see later, if we want to stay young it is important we find an inner balance: it is equally important that we learn how to improve our general health by learning how to eat well. It is the core message of this book. Only by preserving its dynamism and *joie de vivre* will the generation of baby-boomers experience its second youth and make those roaring fifties a reality.

PART TWO
Understand Before You Act

1 What Changes after Fifty

Half a century is both a long and a short time. In fact, it is not very much for a body programmed to live a hundred and twenty years. Having attained maturity, at least twenty-five years of that life should be spent in cruising mode.

It is interesting to ask how our body has evolved and particularly what have been the main changes in its principal functions.

CHANGES TO THE DIGESTIVE MECHANISM

The marks of age are generally considered to be wrinkles, a dry skin, a compacted silhouette, a slightly curved back and a loss of muscle tone. Well, those are the visible parts of the iceberg.

On the inside, a certain number of functions have deteriorated a little. At the cardiovascular level, we know that the vessels have a tendency to harden and clog up, and as far as the heart is concerned, it may occasionally misfire. There may also be some urinary problems and perhaps pains that indicate arthritis has taken up residence in the joints. Long-sightedness makes it necessary to wear glasses to see things close at hand.

In this chorus of minor failures, the digestive tract is not an organ whose performance is often considered, except in connection with the perennial problem of constipation. Notwithstanding this, the digestive system does undergo change, which has consequences as far as the alimentary process is concerned.

The Appetite

With age, our taste buds tend to degenerate. The taste of things therefore changes. As a result, we can become too liberal when using salt, spices and even fat in order to obtain a more distinctive flavour.

The sense of smell may also become less sensitive. Combined with the disruption to our sense of taste, this can only lead to a reduced interest in food due to its perceived blandness. There is thus a risk that certain people will suffer a progressive loss of appetite, leading occasionally to anorexia.

The Digestion

Dental problems, often due to lack of care, can interfere with our chewing action. Studies have shown that if such problems are too often neglected, they can lead to significant changes in our eating habits, and eventually to malnutrition.

As far as the action of the stomach is concerned, the reduced secretion of acids lowers the rate at which proteins (found in meats, fish, eggs, cheeses) are digested, whilst slower gastric evacuation lengthens the process of digestion.

The digestive secretions of the gall bladder and the pancreas also diminish with age, affecting the absorption of nutrients by the body (proteins, carbohydrates and fats) and slowing down the digestive process in the intestine.

Among mineral salts, only the absorption of calcium seems to be affected adversely by these changes. However, this slowing down in the passage of food down the gut will often give rise to the classic problems of constipation, which has to be fought with an appropriate diet (see chapter 7).

The metabolism of nutrients

Proteins

The lean mass of the body - that is to say, its protein mass - diminishes appreciably as the years pass. For those leading a predominantly sedentary lifestyle, this process can starts from the age of twenty-five.

This reduction is due principally to the loss of muscle mass around the bones. It is thought a man will lose twelve kilos (26 lbs) in muscle mass between the ages of twenty-five and seventy-five.

Furthermore, muscle protein is replaced at an ever-decreasing rate as the years go by. In the event of a prolonged confinement in bed, the loss of muscle tissue that ensues can be quite catastrophic.

Fats

In contrast, fatty mass has a tendency to increase with age, with a change to its geographic distribution. It seems to accumulate most readily in the upper part of the body, above the navel and within the abdomen. It is in this region that obesity normally manifests itself.

Conversely, after the age of sixty-five, the levels of cholesterol - even when slightly higher than normal (particularly LDL) - will pose few coronary risks. Paradoxically, it has been noted that low levels of cholesterol (below 1.70gm), which would be considered ideal for a man of thirty-five, can even constitute a risk factor for a man over sixty-five.

Carbohydrates

When a carbohydrate (starch, flour, sugar) has been ingested, the increase in glycaemia (level of glucose or sugar in the blood) causes the pancreas to secrete insulin - the hormone that promotes the passage of glucose into the body cells that have need of the energy it contains.

After the age of sixty, the pancreas become more sluggish and this results in raised sugar levels in the blood over longer periods of time after a meal. Reduced physical activity aggravates the condition, since low muscular activity results in a low burn-up of sugar.

In addition, the body is frequently intolerant to lactose, the carbohydrate of unfermented milk products, because the enzyme lactase that is necessary to digest it is often not secreted by an adult - a state of affairs that is even more likely to occur with an older person.

It will therefore be important to bear these phenomena in mind when deciding which carbohydrates to eat, as we shall see later on.

The elimination of waste products

With the passing of the years, the kidneys can also become less efficient in purifying the blood, resulting in the accumulation of waste products derived from the metabolism of proteins, such as urea and uric acid.

These disruptions to the digestive system are not often well known. It is therefore important to mention them here, for we will see that they help to determine the nutritional options we will discuss later on.

Beyond a certain age, and even more importantly at a certain age, it is generally considered normal to eat less, particularly if physical activity has been markedly reduced. This is a piece of current wisdom that is founded on false premises.

Bearing in mind the changes that result from the reduced efficiency of an ageing alimentary tract, it is necessary in the second half of life to eat normal amounts of food with a high nutritional content.

THE PSYCHOLOGICAL FACTORS

At the beginning of the century, couples willingly had four, six, even ten children. They could then reasonably hope that within the brood there would be some that would achieve adulthood and be able to take care of them in their old age. For in those days, homes for the elderly did not exist and only the family could offer the surroundings necessary for the survival of the grandparents. However, in addition to the relative financial security offered by this arrangement, there was an additional benefit.

The family, which stayed welded together with several generations living in the same house, offered a psychological environment that allowed the third age to blossom.

As a result of the low birth rate and the break-up of families, this situation no longer prevails today. The desire of young couples to be independent, the geographic mobility caused by unemployment, the pokiness of our modern homes and their exorbitant cost, particularly in towns, are all factors that have separated generations from each other. This has led to a very real segregation, in which grandparents live more-or-less alone, seeing few people. As a result, boredom is born together with a certain lack of interest in living, often expressed as a loss of appetite.

Being widowed detracts even more from the pleasure derived from eating. Three out of four people live on their own after the age of seventy-five. The woman who has cooked for others all her life derives little pleasure in doing it just for herself. A man who has been ministered to for so many years by his wife is unlikely suddenly to discover the joys of cooking at the tender age of seventy-five.

Physical handicaps can also be a problem, giving rise to difficulties in obtaining supplies, going shopping, climbing flights of stairs. For some, the inability to drive a car will impose restrictions: instead of going to large supermarkets, they will be obliged to shop in small retail outlets which, apart from being more expensive, are increasingly becoming a rarity.

Going shopping is thus no longer a pleasure. In fact, it becomes a grind - even a trial of endurance. Then you become dependent on others, on your children if they do not live too far away, or your neighbours. Meals-on-wheels furnished by social services are not necessarily the best solution either, for they severely restrict the choice of food available.

Thus we can see that a retirement badly prepared, compounded by health problems and social isolation, can lead to a depressive state which can only aggravate anorexia and lead finally to malnutrition.

In these circumstances, the departure to a retirement home may appear a good solution, since theoretically the meals there are prepared by professionals. Unfortunately, the reality is not so rosy, for often no account is taken of personal preferences and there is little or no choice in the meals to be had. As a result, it has been found that there are many more cases of malnutrition in institutions than are found amongst those who either have remained at home or who live with their family.

FINANCIAL RESOURCES

The precarious nature of their own resources and the lack of financial aid from their children - who themselves are often beset by financial problems - tend to direct retired people to buy food that is cheap and easy to store.

Choice is therefore directed more towards foods containing sugar, foods made from white flour and canned foods - basically foods with a low nutritional content - and at the same time the consumption of meat and fish, rich in protein and iron, is low.

It is necessary therefore to educate these people, showing them how to buy food that is both cheap and rich in proteins, vitamins and mineral salts.

THE MEDICINE CULTURE

A longer life does not reduce the incidence of minor ailments, which modern medicine can alleviate by prescribing an assortment of drugs. Unfortunately, the variety of diseases that exist - whether benign or serious - leads to an excessive consumption of medicines.

Thus for a person who is diabetic, arthritic, constipated and insomniac, a doctor may prescribe four different medicines to relieve each of the four different conditions.

Sometimes the situation is even more complex: for instance, when treating a patient suffering with both Parkinson's disease and hypertension of the arteries.

It should also be remembered that mental disorders account for a significant proportion of prescribed medicines. Of those over eighty years old who find themselves hospitalised, 58% are given psychotropic drugs, of which 38% are neuroleptic and 32% antidepressant. And we know that all these medicines give rise to a pronounced dryness of the mouth, they change perceived taste, reduce salivation and promote constipation.

In addition to regular prescription by the attendant doctor, often prolonged by regular interventions by the specialist, it usual for the elderly to take non-prescribed medicines from time to time in order to calm digestive troubles, constipation or minor aches and pains. This cocktail of medication can aggravate anorexia, lead to digestive troubles, loss of taste, a manifestation of allergies and sometimes feelings of nausea.

What is more, ageing causes the liver and the kidneys to be less efficient. As a result, the elderly have difficulty in metabolising such large quantities of medication and it is not surprising if they often display symptoms of poisoning.

It should also be realised that certain medicines interfere with nutrition by blocking the absorption of iron (stomach emulsions) or vitamins (antibiotics, anti-coagulants and drugs to combat epilepsy). Other medicines if not properly administered can contribute to the loss of mineral salts (diuretics and laxatives), not to mention those that cause weight gain or upset the metabolism of sugars (betablockers or cortisone, for example).

Which all goes to show how much more parsimonious we should be in the prescription of drugs to the elderly, desisting from giving them so-called "comfort medication" to overtax their bodies and perhaps cause nutritional problems that are themselves prejudicial to good health.

2 Nutritional requirements to stay young

RECOGNISE OUR MISTAKES

Before considering how we should feed ourselves, it is important to bear in mind the sort of mistakes people make in their eating habits. Not only do they not eat enough but they also eat badly. And by and large, it is the deficiencies that are most obvious, rather than the excesses.

Early into your fifties, but mainly well beyond that, your diet begins to lack sufficient:

- protein
- fibre
- antioxidants
- iron
- calcium
- water

and have an excess of:

- saturated fats
- sugary foods
- salt
- alcohol.

These several mistakes, which we will examine in detail later on, accelerate the ageing process and, above all, make the constitution of the individual more fragile. They make it more vulnerable to illness and risk undermining its general condition. Sometimes they may even prejudice its longevity.

It is necessary to re-examine a number of generally accepted ideas and modify a certain number of our bad eating habits in order to develop a diet that will maximise our vitality and guard against illness.

If some feel their old eating habits are being called into question and then go on to ask themselves "why should I change at my age?", well perhaps then we should doubt seriously whether they can really benefit from reading this book. Alternatively, if their intention is merely to glean some advice here or there, without taking on board the general thrust of what is said because it will cramp their style too much, then they are likely to be disappointed by the results.

As a method possesses a certain coherence, it should be applied in its entirety: applying a principal in isolation can only result in a very limited beneficial effect.

TRADITION AND LIFESTYLE

French adults, and even more so their elders, are attached to a certain number of traditions and are apparently convinced that there is nothing better than French cooking. This belief should help protect them from the insidious effects of advertising, aimed at encouraging the consumption of industrial food products at the expense of food prepared in the traditional manner.

Rarely do you see a woman of sixty-five eating a sandwich whilst standing in the kitchen. If she is alone, there is little chance she will cook herself an elaborate meal - she will often be satisfied with making do.

It is important we preserve certain rituals associated with a meal, eating at regular times, seated and at rest, and if possible, placing a cloth on the table. A meal should always be one of the great moments of the day - of which there should be at least three. The fourth, afternoon tea, is perhaps more for the retired, since it is often the best time for them to exchange hospitality with others. Eating is a social act and, without doubt, the act of sharing and eating food together always stimulates the appetite.

The important thing is not to remove the social aspect of taking a meal, even when alone, otherwise it runs the risk of becoming slipshod, of progressively losing its interest and leading rapidly to malnutrition.

BEWARE OF DIETS!

After a certain age, there is a tendency to eat less, but particularly to eat badly. As a result, it is wise to mistrust any dietary method that sets out to exclude a large number of foods, as is the case with macrobiotic diets.

Certain illnesses require special dietary precautions. But however suitable they may be at the age of fifty-five, by the age of eighty they may well be useless. This is why there is no cause to worry about an octogenarian with a high cholesterol count, just as it is unreasonable to force a woman of seventy-five to lose weight if she does not have a catastrophic weight problem that really compromises her independence.

If we are put in the position of having to give advice about which foods to eat, it is better to concentrate on what should be eaten rather than insisting on the dishes that should be discarded. By the same token, it is always better to juggle around with the foods preferred by the person seeking advice. You stand the best chance of having your advice followed, if you concentrate on what is allowed and introduce variety to ensure a good dietary balance.

ENERGY INTAKE

In this area there are two aspects to be considered:

1. the energy contained within foodstuffs (normally expressed in calories, of which more later)

2. the daily ration desirable beyond a certain age.

The energy value of food

For a given weight, the fundamental constituents of the food we eat contain different amounts of energy. For instance:

- 1 gram of lipids (fats) contains 9 calories. (In normal conversation we talk about calories, when in fact we are dealing with kilocalories. Though were we to use internationally accepted terms, we should talk about kilojoules, knowing that 1 kilocalorie = 4.8 kilojoules!)

- 1 gram of carbohydrates or sugars produces 4 calories.

- 1 gram of protein produces 4 calories.

- 1 gram of alcohol produces 7 calories.

In addition, there are tables that make it possible to calculate the energy produced by a chosen food.

However, when nutritionists recommend a balanced diet, they are talking about a theoretically desirable diet consisting of:

- carbohydrates (sugars, starches, cereals, flours) making up 50% of the total food intake

- fats 35%

- proteins 15%.

The calculation is always very difficult, perhaps impossible, in that carbohydrates, fats and proteins are often mixed together in the same foodstuff. In addition, the tables that are available only give a theoretical value.

As far as meat is concerned, the proportion of fat can double depending on the piece you cut. Furthermore, the method of cooking can make an appreciable difference to the final energy content. In addition, the calorific intake is profoundly affected by the fibre content of a food and the way it bonds with carbohydrates. It can even be affected by the fibrous content of other foods eaten at the same time. Other substances, like calcium in cheese, can neutralise a part of the energy intake by impeding the total absorption of fats.

In addition, the studies of Reinberg on chronobiology have shown that the energy absorption from foodstuffs - that is to say, the way they are utilised by the metabolism - varies according to the hour of the day and the season considered. Carbohydrates are burned up more easily in the morning and in summer. So it can be seen that the calorific value of a meal is quite relative. In fact you might even say it is nearly always wrong. However, it does allow you to estimate whether someone's diet is more-or-less correct.

Bearing all this in mind, let us then see what sort of energy intake is advisable.

The recommended food intake

Eat Enough

Once and for all, we must sweep away the received notion that because we are not as young as we used to be and are now retired, we can or should eat less.

A notion could not be more mistaken! Older people are as active and sometimes even more active than young adults. What is more, given the fact that their digestive system does not function as well as it used to, causing in a certain slowing down of their metabolism, if they want to be sure of absorbing an adequate quantity of nutrients, they must ensure that they increase the amount of food ingested.

The amount of food they eat must at least maintain the "normal" levels of the past and certainly not be reduced.

Paradoxically, it is during periods of illness that the amount of food eaten should be increased. When things are normal, it is a question of eating at least enough - that is to say, about 2,000 calories a day.

A study of people between the ages of sixty-five and ninety living in Lille, a medium-sized industrial town in northeast France, gave the following figures for energy intake:

	Men	Women
Less than 1,200 kcal	1%	9%
1,200 - 1,600 kcal	9%	35%
1,600 - 2,000 kcal	31%	39%
2,000 - 2,500 kcal	34%	16%
More than 2,500 kcal	25%	1%

It was discovered that many women eat less than 1,600 kcal per day (particularly in the 65-70 and 76-80-year-old groups). But this data includes the calorific value of alcohol consumed by members of the sample group. Taking into consideration only those calories that were ingested as a result of eating proteins, carbohydrates and sugars, the distribution of intake was quite different:

	Men	Women
Less than 1,200 kcal	5%	18%
1,200 - 1,600 kcal	21%	36%
1,600 - 2,000 kcal	36%	39%
2,000 - 2,500 kcal	25%	6%
More than 2,500 kcal	13%	1%

When a diet contains less than 1,600 kcal, and the dietary balance is lacking (which is most often the case when there is no clear understanding of dietary principles), there is always a lack in micronutrients (vitamins, mineral salts and trace elements) and this can have dramatic consequences for an elderly person.

It is currently known that women who are overweight eat less - about 1,500 kcal on average - whilst slim women consume about 2,300 kcal. The statistics show also that widows eat much less (1,400 kcal) than when they lived with their husbands (1,850 kcal).

However, eating more is not such a fantastic solution if the increase in consumption only results in more calories being ingested without improving the quality of the food.

Experiments with animals have also shown that life expectancy can be increased and certain characteristics of old age can be reduced by lowering the energy intake and increasing the nutritional content of food.

Eat well

My advice is that we should eat normally and eat well, choosing foods rich in protein, micronutrients and fibre. Therefore, when selecting our food, our first concern should be to determine its quality. To assist you in this task, we shall now examine nutrients.

3 Different categories of food

To make an informed choice when selecting food, it is imperative we should be familiar with the categories of food available to us and understand fully their various characteristics. In this chapter we shall study these food categories and their various effects.

Macronutrients are present in relatively high concentrations and are expressed in grams. They are:

• water

• proteins

• sugars

• fats

• fibre

• alcohol.

Micronutrients are present in weak concentrations, since they are expressed in milligrams and even micrograms (in millionths of a gram). These are:

• vitamins

• mineral salts

• trace elements.

MACRONUTRIENTS

In addition to their role of providing our bodies with energy, they are synthesised in many different ways to help build and rebuild body cells.

Proteins

These are the organic substances that form the framework of cellular structures in the body. They are derived from animal sources (meat, offal, fish, shellfish, eggs, milk products and cheeses) and vegetable sources (soya, algae, nuts, chocolate, unrefined cereals, pulses such as lentils, beans, chick peas).

A proper intake of protein is essential:

• to build and maintain cellular structures

• to synthesise certain hormones

• to maintain the muscular system

• to make the acids contained in bile.

It is important there should be a balanced intake of protein from both animal and vegetable sources, since they complement one another. The following table shows how this balance may be achieved:

Meal	Foodstuff	Animal Protein	Vegetable Protein
Breakfast	200ml milk	7g	–
	15g cocoa powder	–	5g
	200g bread made with unrefined flour	–	18g
Lunch	150g fish	23g	–
	50g pasta made with unrefined flour	–	5g
Dinner	150g lentils	–	12g
	50g cheese	5g	–
Total		**40g**	**40g**

The ratio of protein mass in the body

If the non-fatty mass constitutes 45% of the weight of an adult at the age of twenty-five, at the age of seventy-five the ratio is no more than 27%. To ensure this situation does not worsen, it is imperative that the daily intake of protein should be about 1g per kilo of body weight (see the table in Appendix 4 at the end of this book). However, this amount should be increased to allow for specific bodily needs: for instance, to combat infection or to heal wounds and bedsores.

A lack of protein will tend to depress the immune system and thus encourage the occurrence of infections or even cancers. Whereas, adding 15g of milk-based protein (found in cheese) to the minimum intake of 1g/kg per day, will help stimulate our immune response.

Can we replace meat?

With age, sometimes we develop a certain dislike for meat, simply because it may be difficult to chew or be too expensive. If this is the case, the animal protein can be replaced with fish, cheese or eggs.

Sheep, pig or beef liver is also a good replacement from time to time, as it is rich in iron and vitamins, is relatively cheap and is easy to chew. Black pudding, when it is not fat, is also rich in protein (16g for every 100g) and in iron (15g).

Milk products cannot completely replace meat (though eggs can), because they do not contain either vitamin B12 or iron.

Do we eat enough protein?

Several studies conducted on people over the age of seventy-five show that 37% of men and 39% of women eat less than 0.80g/kg of protein per day.

Where tests reveal impaired kidney function, it is worthwhile keeping an eye on levels of urea and uric acid in the blood, to see whether the waste products of protein metabolism are building up too much.

On the other hand, even if kidney function is impaired, it is rarely necessary to reduce the amount of protein that is eaten. In fact, it has been concluded that this course of action is useless and does not cause renal function to improve.

Carbohydrates

These are divided into two categories:

- "Simple sugars" like fructose in fruit, galactose in milk, saccharose in cane and beet sugar, lactose in milk or again maltose in beer. They are called "simple" sugars because they are composed of only one or two molecules and require little digestive action before the intestine can absorb them.

- "Complex sugars", composed of starch, which means they require a more complex process of digestion. They are present in all cereals (wheat, maize, rice, rye, barley, oats), tubers (potatoes, yams), roots (carrots, swedes) or pulses (peas, chick peas, beans, lentils, soya).

Hyperglycaemia and hyperinsulinism

All carbohydrates metabolise into glucose and are transported within the body by the bloodstream. Glycaemia can therefore indicate the level of glucose contained in the blood.

On an empty stomach, the glycaemic level is normally 1g of glucose per litre of blood. But after the ingestion of a carbohydrate, the glycaemic level changes (a function of carbohydrates) until it reaches its maximum, which is called the "glycaemic peak". At a certain point, the pancreas secretes a hormone called insulin, which will then promote the passage of glucose from the blood into the muscle tissue as potential energy, or will store it mainly in the liver as glycogen.

Normally, the amount of insulin induced by glycaemia is proportional to the level of glucose in the blood. Often, however, the secretion of insulin is disproportionate. When it is excessive, we talk of hyperinsulinism - a condition that can have many consequences, as we shall see later on.

Beyond a certain age, we encounter two problems connected with the poor assimilation of glucose: hyperglycaemia and hyperinsulinism.

Hyperglycaemia, which occurs frequently after the age of seventy, may reach a level of 1.70g per litre of blood on an empty stomach without there being any cause for alarm. On the other hand, this hyperglycaemia causes hyperinsulinism, which can have unpleasant consequences: reactive hypoglycaemia (fatigue, depression) or weight gain.

Carbohydrates and proteins react chemically with one another, bringing about what has been called the *Maillard Reaction* - something that occurs when cooking foods containing both carbohydrates and proteins. What is more, the chemical compounds that result from this reaction appear to affect tissues that have a slow rate of renewal, such as arteries and the lens of the eye.

The compounds created by the Maillard Reaction accelerate the ageing process and because of this, it is essential that hyperglycaemia (high level of glucose in the blood) should be brought under control.

It is of course important to remember that a carbohydrate is not necessarily a sugar; it is often a starch. In fact, it is thanks to the Maillard Reaction that we obtain crust on our bread and the appetising aroma that goes with it.

Lactose intolerance

Lactose is the sugar found in milk. For it to be assimilated, this molecule must be broken into two by an enzyme lactase, thereby producing glucose and galactose. Apparently, 50% of adults produce insufficient lactase for their requirements and this percentage increases rapidly with age.

This difficulty often translates into diarrhoea (which can occur several hours after digesting milk) but more usually it manifests itself in flatulence and an inflated gut. What is more, it is interesting to note that the accumulation of badly digested lactose can contribute to the formation of cataracts - a telltale sign of old age if ever there was one!

For this reason, if anyone suspects they are intolerant to lactose - which is frequently the case - then they should eliminate from their diet milk products that contain lactose:

• milk (even if skimmed)

• white cheese

• petits-suisse cheeses

• all preparations with a milk base.

However, there are no problems associated with milk products that have lost most or all of their lactose as a result of fermentation, like yoghurts and cheeses.

There are of course commercial preparations on the French market, like "AL 110" milk, which do not contain lactose, but it is possible to take lactase in tablet form or add it to milk products some hours before consuming them.

Beware of sugar!

So-called "simple" sugars, such as saccharose and fructose from fruit, should not make up more than 10% of our daily energy intake. The essential part of this intake should be derived from fruit containing vitamins and mineral salts as well as energy. There is therefore little place for white sugar, which has no nutritional content at all.

And yet the elderly often have a tendency to eat too many sugar products, since they calm anxiety, increase tolerance to pain and are easy to digest. Furthermore, they need no preparation in the kitchen. However, in addition to the fact that sugars increase glycaemia with the consequences we have already seen (hyperinsulinism), they also lower our appetite and so reduce our intake of foods rich in protein and vitamins.

Select carbohydrates with a low glycaemic index (see Part 3 – Chapter 3)

As far as our choice of carbohydrates is concerned, quality should always prevail over quantity.

If we bear in mind the metabolic conditions likely to prevail after a certain age, preference should be given to carbohydrates with a low glycaemic index (below 60). Carbohydrates have been classified in terms of their glycaemic potential, based on the value of pure glucose that has been given a reference figure of 100 (see the table on page 115).

Carbohydrates with a low glycaemic index (below 60) have several advantages, as they:

• give rise to lower glucose levels in the blood

• trigger a reduced secretion of insulin from the pancreas

• limit the compounds generated by the Maillard Reaction

• are rich in vegetable protein

• are rich in fibre

• contain more micronutrients (vitamins, mineral salts, trace elements).

The choice of carbohydrates therefore plays a pivotal role in regulating the ageing process. Choosing carbohydrates with a low glycaemic index as well as reducing or eliminating lactose from your diet are essential steps in realising this goal.

Unfortunately, consumer surveys show clearly that:

- consumption of sugar (saccharose) is too high, making up more than 20% of the energy sourced by the body

- consumption of carbohydrates with a high glycaemic index (white rice, refined white flour, potatoes as opposed to unrefined cereals and pulses) is not only too high, but is continually going up

- fresh milk products (white cheese, milk, etc.) containing lactose, are continually being offered to elderly people, particularly those in institutions.

Fats

For several decades, fats have been the objects of a real psychosis on the part of nutritionists. You only have to look at the United States to see how it has developed into a sort of paranoia. Almost every ill you can think of has been laid at the door of fats at one time or the other. Obesity and cardiovascular disease have been particular favourites. Fortunately this obsession has become less marked in recent years.

Fats are indispensable

Lipids are an essential food for the body because they:

- provide energy in an easily stored form

- are necessary for the formation of cellular membrane and particularly the neurones of the brain

- facilitate the manufacture of hormones and prostaglandin

- transport fat-soluble vitamins (A, D, E and K)

- contribute to the manufacture of bile salts

- are the sole source of essential fatty acids.

The two facets of cholesterol

Cholesterol is not the intruder in the body that we have come to think. It is necessary for ensuring cell membranes remain permeable, for the formation of hormones in the adrenal glands and for the manufacture of vitamin D in the skin.

Contrary to what we are often led to believe, there is no connection between the level of cholesterol in food and the level to be found in the blood. The bulk of cholesterol is, in fact, manufactured by the body in the liver.

Moreover, there is not *one* cholesterol but *several* cholesterols present in varying quantities in a given measure of blood. Details are as follows:

- The overall level of cholesterol in the blood of a young adult, should be less than 2g/l.

- LDL cholesterol - the so-called "bad" cholesterol that has the tendency to deposit on the walls of the arteries obstructing the flow of blood - should be less than 1.3g/l in a young adult.

- HDL cholesterol - the so-called "good" cholesterol that does not settle on the walls of the arteries but actually cleans away the fatty deposits that have collected there. It follows therefore that the higher the level of this substance in the blood, the lower is the risk of a cardiovascular accident or heart attack. Ideally, the level should be above 0.45g/l in the case of a man and above 0.55g/l in the case of a woman.

In fact, what is important is that the ratio between the total level of cholesterol and HDL cholesterol should not exceed 4.5.

The different fats or fatty acids

In food, fats are often found in the form of triglycerides, which after digestion are transformed into fatty acids.

There are three types of fatty acids:

- Saturated fatty acids found in:

    - meat and cooked meats

    - chicken skin

    - full-fat milk products, like butter and cheese

    - eggs

    - palm oil, cabbage palm and copra.

They increase the total amount of cholesterol and LDL cholesterol in the blood and tend to encourage the deposit of fat that can narrow the arteries.

• Polyunsaturated fatty acids, having:

- a vegetable origin - oils derived from walnut, hazelnut, almond, sunflower, maize, soya, rapeseed and peanut, as well as vegetable margarine

- an animal origin - fish oils.

The fatty acids contribute to lowering the total cholesterol level, but unfortunately, they also lower HDL cholesterol.

• Mono-unsaturated fatty acids, found principally in:

- olive oil

- goose and duck fat

- foie-gras

- cocoa.

These fatty acids lower the total level of cholesterol and LDL cholesterol and may even increase "good" cholesterol. This is the reason they may be given an important place in our daily ration of fat.

• Fat supplies

Several surveys conducted in 1988-1989 showed that fat accounted for 35% of the total diet of people over the age of sixty, whilst nutritionists maintain that it should not exceed 30%. However, it is not so much the quantity of fat consumed that is important but rather the quality.

The only valid reason for reducing the total quantity of fats consumed is the prevention of certain types of cancer. In fact, the incidence of cancers or the prostate and colon are highest if the daily diet of fat exceeds 40%.

• Saturated fatty acids

- Eating meat every day should be avoided; three or four times a week is sufficient for the proper supply of protein, iron and vitamin B12, if alternated with chicken dishes, eggs and fish. Naturally, only the leanest cuts of meat should be selected.

- Milk products should be semi-skimmed or fully skimmed, bearing in mind that the difference between a natural yoghurt with 1.2% fat and a low-fat yoghurt with 0.3% fat, is almost insignificant.

- The higher the calcium content of a cheese the harder it is for its saturated fats to be absorbed through the gut. So we should not cut back on these types of cheese, particularly as we know they contain no lactose and are rich in protein.

- Eggs also contain saturated fatty acids and cholesterol. But all this is largely counterbalanced - not to say, largely neutralised - by the presence of lecithin. No reason then, to exclude them from your diet.

- As far as palm oil is concerned, although its merits have long been extolled because of its vegetable origins, it should be avoided as much as possible because it is certainly one of the worst fats. It is to be found in most biscuits and industrial pastries. It can even hide behind the vague title of "vegetable oil" in the list of ingredients used by the food industry. So try and select foods that clearly specify the oil that has been used, whether olive or sunflower.

Polyunsaturated or mono-unsaturated fatty acids

Olive oil is the overall champion in the league of "good oils". It can therefore be used - even to excess - providing it is classified as "Virgin" and is from the first cold pressing. All this information will be found on the label if the oil meets these criteria.

Olive oil is in fact the pillar of the world-famous Mediterranean (or more precisely, Cretan) diet, which offers its followers the best protection against cardiovascular disease. But as it does not contain all the nutrients we need (particularly essential fatty acids), it is advisable to use sunflower oil as well, particularly for seasoning. However, it should be remembered that vegetable oils in general are chemically modified in the cooking process and can thus develop a cardiovascular toxicity that in their natural state they do not possess.

When cooking, it is better to use olive oil or goose fat, as they remain more stable when subjected to heat.

So-called "essential" fatty acids

There are two fatty acids that our diet must contain, since they are as indispensable as vitamins.

• Linoleic acid

This is found in sunflower and corn oil. The body of an adult contains sufficient reserves of this substance to last for sixty days. An elderly person, however, needs to have it included in their daily intake of food - something that unfortunately is not always the case.

Its absence leads to cellular problems affecting the skin, the mucous tissue and the endocrine glands, but also leads to the risk of possible arterial lesions.

• Alphalinolenic acid

The daily intake should be 2g per day, but on average elderly people consume less than 250mg per day. This is eight times less than the recommended intake. What is more, 20% of the elderly consume no alphalinolenic acid at all.

It is to be found in rapeseed and walnut oil, as well as hazelnuts, almonds and even butter. A lack of this substance can cause changes in the cellular membrane, notably in the brain - leading to memory problems and learning difficulties, as well as causing lesions in the retina, which will radically affect vision.

Other indispensable fatty acids

• DHA

This fatty acid plays a structural role in the formation and maintenance of brain tissue. In theory, the body can manufacture it from alphalinolenic acid in the liver. But this transformation is no longer possible in elderly people, where certain enzymes no longer function very well.

• EPA

This fatty acid has an essential role in helping to prevent cardiovascular accidents, since it

- lowers the level of triglycerides
- causes the blood to flow more easily, preventing the formation of clots leading to thrombosis
- contributes to the lowering of cholesterol levels.

To have an adequate intake of these two fatty acids, it is only necessary to eat 100g of fish three or four times a week. Any fish will do, but salmon, sardines and mackerel are particularly good.

ENERGY-FREE MACRONUTRIENTS

The benefits of fibre

Fibre has long been ignored because it has no energy value. We know today, however, that it has a very important nutritional role to play, particularly as a regulator in many metabolic reactions.

Insoluble fibre

This group covers cellulose, the majority of the hemi-celluloses and woody fibres. It is found principally in fruit, vegetables and legumes (pulses).

By absorbing water and increasing their volume like a sponge, insoluble fibre helps faeces become moist and bulky and make an important contribution to the fight against constipation that affects many elderly people. In addition, they inhibit the formation of stones in the gall bladder and help prevent the formation of cancers in the colon and rectum.

Soluble fibre

This group covers pectin (fruit), gum (legumes), algae (seaweed) and certain hemi-celluloses (barley, oats).

Soluble fibre forms a thick gel by absorbing a high quantity of water and it alters the absorption of carbohydrates and fats. As a result, it reduces hyperglycaemia and helps control hyperinsulinism, a condition that afflicts many in the second half of their life, and it also helps stabilise diabetes should it develop.

In addition, soluble fibre helps reduce the level of cholesterol and triglycerides in the blood, thereby contributing to the prevention of cardiovascular disease.

The downside of fibre

By fermenting in the intestines, fibre contributes to the generation of gas, subjecting the gut to internal pressure and giving rise to unpleasant abdominal pain. This is very often the case with those making a rapid transition - from one day to the next - from a diet containing little fibre to one that has a lot. These problems can be particularly evident with people over sixty, who have fragile intestines and suffer with spasmodic colitis.

To avoid troubles of this kind, those who have eaten little fibre in the past, should gradually increase their portion of fibre by about 5g a week, so that the large intestine can have time to adjust and the intestinal flora can adapt to the changed environment in the gut. Even a person suffering with colitis or diverticulosis should eat fibre, alternating between raw and cooked fibre to reduce the likelihood of irritation.

At the beginning, it is possible to limit pressure on the gut and reduce colic pains by taking medicinal clay or charcoal, or having recourse to antispasmodic medication.

In the past, phytic acid from cereals was accused of preventing the absorption of calcium. Some even claimed that bread made from unrefined flour was decalcifying. More recent studies have shown that nothing of the sort happens, particularly if the bread is made with yeast and, following traditional methods, kneading is slow.

Likewise, it is incorrect to think that fibre can interfere with the absorption of vitamins, mineral salts and trace elements.

How to eat fibre each day

The ideal ration of fibre each day is about 30 to 40g. Statistical studies on the third age now show that average consumption is less than 20g a day and that this amount reduces as people get older.

Age in Years	60-64	65-69	70-74	75-79	+80
Men	20g	17g	14g	13g	9g
Women	15g	17g	19g	17g	14g

It can be seen here that consumption of fibre declines mainly amongst men. This can only encourage constipation and the development of cancers in the digestive tract.

To ensure that an adequate quantity of fibre is consumed, we can easily incorporate foods containing fibre into our daily menu, as follows (see also the table in Appendix 4 at the end of the book):

Breakfast	Lunch and Dinner	Snacks
Fruit	Raw vegetables	Fresh fruit
Cereals	Vegetable soup	Dried fruit (prunes apricots, figs)
Wholewheat bread	Pulses	Wholewheat biscuits
Crackers rich in fibre	Unrefined foods (rice, pasta, semolina)	Oleaginous fruit, (almonds, walnuts, hazelnuts)
Sugar-free jam	Salads	Sugar-free jam
	Wholewheat bread Stewed fruit	

The benefits of drinking

More than two-thirds of our body is made up of liquids. Proper hydration is therefore essential for the body to function properly. It should also be remembered that even minimal dehydration can have a detrimental effect on health.

The elderly do not drink enough

The risk of dehydration increases with age for the following reasons:

• The sensation of thirst is reduced and more sluggish, leading easily to dehydration. It is therefore wise to drink regularly during the course of the day, anticipating the need to drink.

• Some people have the tendency to reduce their intake of liquids in order to avoid urinating, particularly at night.

- Others who have lost their mobility, prefer not to ask for a drink for fear of disturbing those upon whom they depend.

- Reduced sensitivity of the kidneys to anti-diuretic hormones results in poor regulation of urine volume.

- Certain diuretic treatments, when badly administered, can result in a significant loss of liquids.

The consequences of dehydration are important:

- Tiredness increases: for each 1% loss of water, the body loses 10% of its muscular strength. Thus, a person of 60 kilos who loses 1.2 litres of liquid, whether by drinking too little or urinating too much, will find muscular strength reduced by 20%.

- There is an increase of uric acid in the blood, which can lead to the formation of kidney stones.

- There is an increased production of stools, which will be hard and difficult to evacuate.

- The skin will become dry and age more quickly, producing more wrinkles.

All these problems can gain momentum in a quite dramatic way should the patient be suffering with diarrhoea or should fever increase transpiration. On a more mundane level, living in an environment that is far too hot can have the same result.

The prevention of dehydration

Each day, our body loses about 2.4 litres of liquid in the following manner:

- 100ml in faeces

- 1,400ml in urine

- 500ml through vapour expelled during breathing

- 400ml through sweat (and much more in the case of high temperatures).

About 1 litre is absorbed by the body from food. So, to bring the water content of the body back into balance, we need to drink about 1.4 litres of liquid a day. This can be achieved by drinking water, either from the tap or from a bottle of mineral water. However, all the liquids absorbed during the day make their contribution:

- coffee or chicory

- tea

- tisane (as long as it is not diuretic)

- thick or clear soups

- milk (if there is no intolerance to lactose)

- soya juice (incorrectly called soya "milk")

- squeezed fruit juices

- wine

- beer.

On the other hand, it will be necessary to avoid drinking:

- sodas, colas, lemonades and industrially produced fruit juices, which all contain too much sugar

- so-called "light" drinks, too rich in phosphor, which lead to a loss of calcium.

When should we drink?

To avoid the dilution of gastric juices, which become less abundant as we get older, it is advisable not to drink too much either before or during a meal (two glasses should suffice).

On the other hand, it is necessary to drink regularly between meals. In the case of those who tend to snack, a conscious effort should be made to ensure dining is systematic. For people who are never thirsty, drinking a glass of water several times a day should be considered as important as taking a medicine.

The 1.4 litres of liquid that need to be drunk during the course of a day could be made up as follows:

- On waking   0.15 litres (water or fresh fruit juice)

- Breakfast   0.25 litres (skimmed milk, tea or coffee)

- About 10am   0.15 litres (water)

- Lunch   0.20 litres (wine/water)

- About 3pm   0.15 litres (water)

- Snack   0.15 litres (tea or tisane)

- Dinner   0.20 litres (wine/water)

- Bedtime   0.15 litres (tisane or water)

On the other hand, it should not be forgotten that eating salty food increases the amount of water that should be drunk, as does excessive sweating caused by high temperatures or fever. In the case of physical exercise, it is very important to drink before, during and after it takes place.

Alcoholic drinks

Beer

It may be drunk during meals. In which case, the amount should not exceed 0.60 litres per day. It should not be drunk on an empty stomach, to avoid the risk of inducing hypoglycaemia. For this reason alone, it is perhaps better to drink beers containing no alcohol.

Wine

Numerous studies have shown that the consumption of two to three glasses of wine per day is a very effective way of preventing cardiovascular disease. In addition, the polyphenols contained in wine have a major anti-oxidising effect, which enables them to combat free radicals and undermine the ageing process in the body.

Red wines with a significant amount of tannin are also very rich in minerals and trace elements, particularly iron. Certain white wines on the other hand should be avoided, because of their diuretic properties.

MICRONUTRIENTS

Micronutrients such as vitamins, mineral salts and trace elements, act as chemical catalysts for the macronutrients such as proteins, carbohydrates and fats. In effect, they ensure the proper functioning of our "metabolic factory", by promoting the assimilation of energy-giving substrates.

Their presence in proper quantities is indispensable to ensure that the human body is able to function correctly, stay in good health and not become tired.

In Western countries, where there tends to be an overabundance of food, there are no longer any signs of major nutritional deficiencies like scurvy or beriberi. On the other hand, there are quite a few signs of minor nutritional deficiencies, which not only accelerate the process of ageing but also render the human organism much more vulnerable to illness.

An inadequate supply of micronutrients has two causes. First of all, it comes as a result of a badly thought-out diet - principally the result of bad eating habits where meals are no longer varied and always consist of the same foods.

The other reason is that food produced in industrialised nations is often deficient in micronutrients, because of the stress placed on:

- intensive farming methods, dedicated exclusively to increasing productivity by making massive use of chemical fertilisers, pesticides, insecticides and weed killers

- harvesting before the crops have matured

- protracted transport and storage times

- excessive refining (flour dressing, bleaching)

- widespread use of preservatives

- inadequate food preparation

- poorly chosen cooking or reheating methods.

Antioxidants

Principal among these, are:

• vitamin A (and particularly its forerunner, betacarotene)

• vitamin C

• vitamin E

• selenium

• zinc

• copper

• polyphenols.

Their role consists of trapping free radicals which, we need to remind ourselves constantly, are largely involved in the ageing process of body cells in general and brain cells in particular. It is probable that they are also involved in both Parkinson's and Alzheimer's disease.

However, they also play an important role in diseases that frequently occur after the age of fifty, particularly:

• cardiovascular disease

• cancers

• immune deficiencies, the source of infections

• inflammations and sclerosis

• cataracts

• diabetes.

We know that free radicals contribute indirectly to the death of body cells (see Appendix 2 - *Understanding the ageing process)*. It is therefore important that food should contain antioxidants in significant quantities. Studies conducted on those over sixty have shown that the intake of antioxidants is well below what is required.

Unfortunately, there is no laboratory test currently available to measure antioxidants in the body. Measurement of vitamin C in the blood is still rare.

FOODS RICH IN ANTIOXIDANTS

Vitamin E	Vitamin C	Betacarotene	Copper
Wheatgerm oil	Wild Rose hip	Raw carrot	Oysters
Corn oil	Blackcurrants	Watercress	Veal liver
Soya oil	Parsley	Spinach, Sorrel	Sheep's liver
Sunflower oil	Kiwi fruit	Mango	Mussels
Groundnut oil	Broccoli	Melon	Cocoa powder
Rape seed oil	Sorrel	Apricot	Ox liver
Olive oil	Raw peppercorn	Broccoli	Wheatgerm
Peanut oil	Tarragon	Peach	Haricot beans
Wheatgerm	Green cabbage	Tomato	Hazelnuts
Hazelnuts	Watercress	Orange	Dried peas
Almonds	Red cabbage	Dandelion	Oats
Germinated	Lemon	Chervil	Walnuts
cereals	Orange	Parsley	Brains
Walnuts, peanuts			
Wild rice			

Vitamin A	Selenium	Zinc	Polyphenols
Cod liver oil	Oysters	Oysters	Wine
Animal liver	Chicken liver	Dried peas	Grape pips
Butter	Ox liver	Duck liver	Green tea
Cooked egg	Fish	Brewer's yeast	Olive oil
Fresh apricot	Egg	Dried beans	Onions
Cheese	Mushrooms	Kidneys	Apples
Salmon	Onions	Eel	
Full milk	Wholemeal bread	Lentils	
Sardines	Brown rice	Meat	
Crème fraîche	Lentils	Wholemeal bread	
	Brains		

A few highly specialised laboratories have nevertheless perfected tests for general use. But apart from the fact that in France they are only available in major centres like Paris and Lyon, these tests are not subsidised by the health service.

As modern food is deficient in antioxidants, we might be tempted to ask whether we should supplement our diet with antioxidant tablets manufactured by the pharmaceutical industry. Nothing could be more unwise! It would be to forget that vitamins and trace elements do not exist in isolation: for when they occur naturally in foodstuffs, they do so together with other nutrients that facilitate their assimilation. Moreover, it is not easy to administer the correct dose of synthetic nutrients, as more often than not it can be either too little or too much - in which case, the effects can be more harmful than the ill we attempt to correct.

This is the reason we should be very cautious about the use of "food supplements", as no study to date has shown that they can satisfactorily make up what is missing in our regular diet. It would seem rather that to be effective, micronutrients should be contained in a natural "living" substance. Furthermore, we should be more concerned with supplying antioxidants in sufficient quantities, by introducing the appropriate bias into our daily diet.

This is how we could construct a daily menu to ensure a good provision of antioxidants:

Breakfast	Lunch	Snack	Dinner
Fresh Orange Juice	Oysters	Hazelnuts, Almonds, Dried Apricots	Grated Carrots + Olive Oil
2 Kiwis	Veal Liver, Broccoli and Lentils	Green Tea	Salmon and Whole Rice
Wholemeal Bread + Butter	Yoghurt and Brewer's yeast		Watercress Salad
Chocolate Skimmed milk	Glass of Wine		Walnut Cheese
			Glass of Wine

Other Micronutrients

Vitamin B9 or Folic Acid

Vitamin B9 is necessary for the metabolism of proteins and manufacture of body cells. Several studies show that people over sixty are largely deficient in this micronutrient.

This deficiency has several causes:

• a general imbalance in the diet of older people

• resulting infections

• medication, notably in the form of:

>   Bactrim (sulphamide)
>
>   Teriam and Prestole (diuretics)
>
>   Dihydan and Mysoline (anti-epileptics)
>
>   Barbiturates
>
>   Questran (anti-hypocholesterolaemic)
>
>   Glucophage, Stagid (anti-diabetic)
>
>   Furadantine (urinary antiseptic).

• excessive consumption of alcoholic drinks: one litre of wine or 80g of pure alcohol are sufficient to cause a deficiency.

The following symptoms indicate a vitamin B9 deficiency:

• tiredness

• depression

• memory problems

• insomnia

• mental confusion

• altered general state.

Unfortunately, these problems are fairly widespread and, when identified, are more often than not ascribed to the age of the patient and prescribed for with medication (anti-depressants and neuroleptics) although they merely manifest a vitamin deficiency.

It is also quite difficult to reach the recommended daily ration of 300 micrograms of vitamin B9.

Details of the relative concentrations of vitamin B9 in various foods are as follows:

FOODS RICH IN VITAMIN B9

(micrograms per 100g of food)

Brewer's yeast	500 to 1,500
Liver	30 to 80
Oysters	240
Soya Grains	220
Watercress	170 to 320
Fennel	110
Green Vegetables	50 to 110
Dry Vegetables	35 to 130
Wholemeal Bread	40 to 60
Kidneys	30 to 60
Cheese	5 to 60
Milk	50
Haddock	50
Fruit, Carrots	10 to 30
Chocolate	10

It should be remembered that folic acid is very fragile and can easily be destroyed by light, heat and oxidants. All these factors conspire to ensure that anything up to 60% of the initial value of the vitamin is lost. In fact, subjecting the vitamin to a cooking temperature of 110°C for 10 minutes will ensure that 65% of it is destroyed.

Vitamin B6

This micronutrient is necessary for the good functioning of numerous enzymes involved in the metabolism of proteins.

Its lack in the general population and particularly the elderly is significant (8%). Here again, the problem is that the symptoms are rather commonplace and do not elicit particular attention:

• irritability

• tiredness

• vertigo

• nausea

• oily skin

• fondness for sweets.

After all, how many doctors consider a possible deficiency in vitamin B6 when they examine an elderly person who is tired, depressive, irritable and who has a pronounced weakness for sweet things?

To obtain the necessary daily 2mg of B6, it is necessary to seek out the foods that contain significant amounts:

FOODS RICH IN VITAMIN B6

(mg per 100g of food)

Dried Brewer's yeast	5 to 10
Wheatgerm	1 to 5
Soya Germ	1 to 2
Liver (Sheep or Veal)	1.2
Wholemeal Bread	0.5
Dry Vegetables	0.5

Vitamin B6 is also fragile and can be destroyed by:

• light

• refining (the dressing of flour can cause a 75% loss)

• psychotropic medication

• alcohol abuse.

Vitamin D

This vitamin plays an essential role in the absorption of calcium, leading to the strengthening and renewal of our bones.

There are two sources of vitamin D:

1. food

2. skin which, as a result of the action of the sun, is capable of synthesising it.

Exposing the palms of the hands to the sun for fifteen minutes, three days per week between 11am and 2pm, is all that is necessary to obtain the required amount of vitamin D. But unfortunately, many people over the age of seventy do not go out or systematically avoid sitting in the sun. As a result, they run the risk of having a deficiency in vitamin D.

A lack of vitamin D in the elderly often results in osteomalacia (the equivalent of rickets in children), which translates into the rapid development of pain. Here again, it does not follow logically that, when confronted by an elderly person who suddenly has more difficulty in getting around, a diagnosis of vitamin D deficiency should automatically follow. At a more advanced stage of the illness, the doctor may however notice on his X-ray plate characteristic fissures in the bones of the pelvis.

Treatment with vitamin D is soon effective. However, the best way not to develop a deficiency is to eat the following foods regularly and to expose the body to the sun on every possible occasion.

FOODS RICH IN VITAMIN D

Cod liver oil	Mushrooms
Tuna	Pork
Sardine	Chicken
Egg yolk	Animal liver

Vitamin B1

This micronutrient is indispensable for the formation of enzymes that facilitate the breaking down and assimilation of carbohydrates. It also plays an important role in the functioning of the nervous system.

And yet the refined products of our modern diet, like sweet pastries and biscuits, are very poor in vitamin B1. This is more important for people over sixty, as statistics show that 80% of them suffer with deficiencies in vitamin B1.

Apart from deficiencies caused by poor diet, a lack of vitamin B1 is also encouraged by:

• poor intestinal absorption

• diabetes

• too many refined carbohydrates

• diuretics

• fever

• excessive consumption of alcoholic drinks.

A lack of vitamin B1 results in:

• tiredness

• irritability

• memory lapses

• depression

• loss of appetite

• muscular weakness and pain

• constipation.

The 1.5mg necessary each day is to be found in the following foods:

FOODS RICH IN VITAMIN B1

(mg per 100g of food)

Brewer's Yeast	2 to 35
Wheatgerm	0.2 to 3
Wholemeal bread	0.5
Lentils	0.1 to 0.3
Haricots beans	0.1 to 0.3
Kidneys, liver	0.2 to 0.5
Other meats	0.1 to 0.4

But as always, this vitamin is also very fragile and will be partially destroyed:

• by heat (boiling in water or sterilising conserves)

• an excess of alcohol

• certain medications (intestinal preparations, antibiotics, laxatives).

Calcium

Calcium is a mineral salt that is particularly important in the second half of our lives, as its assimilation is indispensable for limiting osteoporosis. The minimum daily intake is 1.5g. However, people in the menopause absorb less than 0.8g per day.

It has several functions:

• maintaining the integrity of the skeleton

• assisting muscular contraction

• reducing arterial tension

• probably offering protection against cancer of the colon.

For an adult under fifty, daily intake should be 1,000mg: for adults over fifty, this should be increased to 1,500mg, particularly for a woman who is vulnerable to osteoporosis (see Part 3 – Chapter 6). For calcium to be correctly bonded to the bones, vitamin D should be present in adequate quantities.

FOODS RICH IN CALCIUM

(mg per 100g of food)

Brewer's yeast	2,000
Gruyere cheese	1,200
Wheatgerm	0.2 to 3
Other cheeses	800 to 1,000
Prunes	800
Sardines with bones	400
Condensed milk	300
Eggs	300
Parsley, Watercress	200
Dried fruit	200
Natural yoghurt	170
White cheese	125

DRINKS RICH IN CALCIUM

(mg per 100g of food)

Milk	1,000
Mineral water (Vittel)	600
Spring water (Vittel)	200
Hard water from Parisian tap	100

Calcium in milk products and mineral waters is much more easily absorbed by the body than is calcium from a vegetable source. Absorption is maximised when it is spread over three or four meals and for those over fifty, ideally a milk product should be eaten at each of the three main daily meals.

Those suffering from a high cholesterol level who wish to protect themselves from cardiovascular disease can eat milk products with a 0% fat content that will contain the same quantity of calcium as their full-fat equivalents.

Magnesium

An adequate daily ration of 400mg is essential, because magnesium:

• is involved in the action of more than 300 enzymes

• plays a major role in muscular contraction

• is involved in the build-up of bone mass

• prevents infections by stimulating the immune response system

• reduces the level of cholesterol and triglycerides in the blood.

A lack of magnesium leads to the following disturbances in the body:

• cardiac problems: coronary spasms, uneven rhythm

• greater vulnerability to stress

• muscular trembling, cramp.

Statistics show that 70 to 80% of people over sixty have a daily intake below the recommended level - a situation that can be aggravated by a poorly controlled diabetic condition, an over-indulgence in refined carbohydrates, stress and alcoholism.

Magnesium levels in the blood can be easily verified.

FOODS RICH IN MAGNESIUM

(mg per 100g of food)

Winkles	420
Wheatbran	420
Cocoa	420
Wheatgerm	340
Soya grain	250
Almonds	250
Brewer's yeast	230
Haricot beans	170
Peanuts	170
Walnuts	150
Wholemeal bread	150
Lentils	100
Mineral water (Vittel)	120
Mineral water (Evian)	20

Potassium

A daily diet of 1,000mg is necessary to protect against arterial hypertension and cramp.

With older people, certain factors can make the effects of a deficiency worse, such as an excessive use of laxatives, diuretic treatments or diarrhoea.

FOODS RICH IN POTASSIUM

(mg per 100g of food)

Brewer's yeast	1,600
Dried apricots	1,500
Lentils	1,500
Haricot beans	1,300
Split peas	1,000
Prunes, dates	1,000
Almonds, hazelnuts	600
Mushrooms	600
Walnuts	600
Artichokes	400
Bananas	400
Chocolate (+70% cocoa)	400

Iron

Iron stimulates the immune system and enters the structure of haemoglobin, facilitating the take up of oxygen by the blood.

A lack of iron produces the following symptoms:

• pallor

• tiredness

• feeling cold, cold extremities

• palpitations

• breathlessness

• difficulty in swallowing (dysphagia)

- reduction in intellectual faculties

- increased risk of infection.

In the case of influenza, lung or urinary infection accompanied by fever, the elderly patient will be forced to take refuge in bed (particularly if over eighty years old). It is a situation that can deteriorate rapidly, due to a lack of appetite and dehydration, into something much more worrying, particularly if the patient is confined to bed for longer than expected.

An iron deficiency can easily be revealed by a blood test.

In addition to poor diet contributing to a lack of iron in the blood, there are other factors that may lie at the root of the condition:

- visible or hidden haemorrhaging, sometimes caused by an hiatus

- hernia

- gastritis

- excessive use of aspirin or anti-inflammatory drugs

- haemorrhoids

- polyp in the colon, colic or rectal cancer

- urinary problems (cystitis, cancer of the bladder)

- too much tea or anti-acid medication

- deficiency of vitamin C.

To maintain the correct level of iron in the blood, 15mg should be consumed each day.

It is important to remember that there are two type of iron:

- *heminic iron*, animal in origin, easily absorbed through the intestine

- *non-heminic iron*, vegetable in origin, which is less easily absorbed. Unfortunately, we cannot hope to absorb sufficient iron from a vegetable source to meet our bodily requirements.

FOODS RICH IN IRON

(mg per 100g of food)

Black pudding	18
Mussels	18
Brewer's yeast	18
Cocoa powder	18
Liver (pork, beef)	10
Dried vegetables	10
Ox tongue	7
Oysters	7
Veal liver	6
Dried apricots, dates	6
Beef	4
Turkey	4
Kidneys	4
Dried figs	4
Almonds, hazelnuts	4
Lamb, pork	3
Eggs, sausages	2
Tuna, sardines	2

Chrome

Chrome plays an essential role in the metabolism of the body, because it improves tolerance to glucose by assisting the action of insulin. That is to say, it is important for a person suffering from hyperinsulinism. It also has the advantage of lowering "bad" cholesterol and raising the level of the "good".

FOODS RICH IN CHROME

Egg yolk	Brewer's yeast
Wheatgerm	Watercress
Beetroot	Liver
Mushrooms	Kidney

A deficiency in chrome will aggravate the following conditions:

• hyperinsulinism

• diabetes

• cataracts

• atheromas

• obesity.

EAT WELL AND STAY YOUNG

PART THREE

Our Plan of Campaign:
act with full knowledge of the facts

1 Strategy for Staying Fit

As all sportsmen will tell you, performance depends on two inseparable factors: the physical and the mental, the body and the spirit. If you have one without the other, the results are disappointing. You need both. However, when you deal with one, you deal with the other. The synergy is total. It is what we are going to do with our programme: tune up the machine and boost the morale of the pilot!

BEAT FATIGUE

The various aspects of fatigue

Fatigue or tiredness is a very vague all-inclusive term, used in general conversation to indicate a lack of form.

There are several types of fatigue:

- Real fatigue, which is due to physical exhaustion. It is a passing physiological state, due to the exhaustion of energy reserves intended for the muscles. Weakness and pain cause the subject to cease his endeavours. But a few hours of rest, a good night's sleep, and everything is all right again.

- The other type of fatigue, called asthenia by doctors, is much more subtle. As you would expect, it is not a normal condition and its causes are often hidden. Technically it is called a morbid state, closer to lassitude and overwork, where the physical and mental causes are interwoven.

This mixture of tiredness and lassitude can manifest itself in many different ways, all of which can be more-or-less apparent:

- a general appearance of poor health: weakness, loss of weight, sweating, waxy colour of the skin

- a reduction in physical tone, resulting in feelings of exhaustion at the slightest effort

- sleeping problems: difficulty in getting to sleep; waking up in the middle of the night often with some manifestation of pain; feeling tired on waking

- decreased intellectual performance: memory lapses, difficulties in concentrating

- feelings of anxiety coupled with pressure on the chest

- character problems: uncontrolled emotional responses, irritability, aggressiveness, withdrawal symptoms

- digestive problems: nausea, anorexia

- problems with the senses: vertigo, headaches, ringing in the ears, opaque vision

- sexual problems: lowered libido, impotence

- lack of drive: increased inhibition, disinterest, depression.

In the face of these symptoms of fatigue, it is important that we remain vigilant in the knowledge that behind these apparently banal signs there may lurk something more serious. Simple investigative procedures, like taking blood samples, X-rays, or even scanning with ultrasound, can help to resolve problems before they have a chance of developing into something more serious.

Causes of fatigue

Overwork

It comes about as a result of excessive effort. It can be:

- physical: as a result of intense professional, housekeeping, gardening or sporting activity

- sensory: living in an environment that is far too noisy

- mental or intellectual.

In fact the "machine" works well, but we ask too much of it. For example, some sixty-year-olds think they can carry on as they did when they were thirty. They have to be reminded that their bodies no longer have the same potential for work and they should learn to divide up their tasks, taking their time and pausing occasionally for a rest.

At the age of seventy, there are men who continue to occupy a respected position in their business, directing it with energy and determination for at least twelve hours a day. However, even these "Errol Flynns of the management world" eventually receive their due warnings, which unfold classically into three phases:

- the alarm phase, with the onset of tiredness, insomnia, anxiety and irritability

- the agitated phase, where for lack of sleep, the patient feels overwhelmed and instead of concentrating on the essentials, he loses himself in useless details, refusing to delegate. Headaches and various pains follow, particularly in the spinal column

- the phase of collapse, which arrives brutally with an attack of arterial hypertension, a stroke or worst of all, a myocardial infarction or heart attack.

- it is in this way that those who pay no heed to the first danger signal of fatigue are finally brought to account. Beyond the age of sixty, we must learn to moderate our lifestyle and "lift our foot off the throttle" when necessary.

Fatigue linked to the abuse of medication

With age, we often become bulimic with regard to our medication. A hypochondriac is asleep in each and every one of us, because we have this naïve belief that for each small ill, the beneficent pharmaceutical industry has concocted a particular medicine for its relief.

It must be said that fifty years ago, when we hurt ourselves, had a sore throat, a small cough or a nagging pain, we expected all would be put right with the simple remedy of a teaspoon of honey, a gentle cup of tea and above all, rest. Later, with the rapid advance of science, the myth of the miracle-pill was born. But what is often forgotten, is that on the back of a few hundred active molecules, there are 36,000 registered medicines. Were these products merely trying to be crowned "wonder drug of the year", then the only ones to suffer would be the National Health Service and our pockets. However, the tragedy is that the chemical substances contained in these medications often do more harm than good.

First of all, there is a problem of determining the right dose. All these medications are conceived for young adults. On the other hand, after the age of fifty, the sensitivity of the body is more pronounced. A few milligrams too many can unleash undesirable effects.

In addition, as the years accumulate, the kidneys and the liver begin to function in an unpredictable way. The prescribed medicinal dose may either be too weak, because a lack of enzymes in the blood will limit its effect, or excessive, because an accelerated metabolism will enhance its concentration in the blood and render it toxic.

Apart from the potentially dangerous effects of taking too many medicines, some of them can be responsible for fatigue, as with:

- betablockers prescribed for hypertension of the arteries, irregular heartbeat or angina

- diuretics

- neuroleptics and tranquillisers that can transform certain people into complete "zombies" (which in certain homes for the elderly is the desired result)

- hypnotic drugs to sleep better, which when taken in excess cause the patient to sleep better by day than by night

- antihistamines taken for allergies (asthma, eczema) and skin irritations

- laxatives, which often lead to dehydration and a loss of potassium.

Mental fatigue

This condition is mainly the result of emotional problems - such as anxiety and depression - which become associated with behavioural problems of aggression and irritability, leading to poor performance (particularly at work). This state is probably the result of stress - a condition that appears when the organism is exposed to new, aggressive stimulation from the world outside. The body must then develop behavioural and metabolic response reactions to adapt to the new conditions.

However, we must distinguish between "good stress" and "bad stress". Good stress is caused by great joy; it is a positive emotion brought on by good news. Except that now, what formerly made you jump with joy and gave you that added impetus to launch yourself into the hurly-burly of life with renewed enthusiasm, now tends to upset your balance to the point that it makes you feel physically exhausted. Too many people over fifty become comfortably ensconced in a well-regulated humdrum existence, where any novelty - even a positive one! - is experienced as a mental and bodily invasion with which they are unable to cope because they lack the necessary suppleness to adapt.

We will see later on in this chapter how we can go about maintaining an open and dynamic spirit, to ensure that we do not react negatively to positive events.

Bad stress is a genuine aggression, experienced as an attack on the integrity of the individual. It creates a very real feeling of "distress". There is a significant quantity of bad stress, which can have different effects according to type, individual sensitivity or occurrence. It is clear that if a husband has been ill for many years and treated as a lost cause by all his doctors, his demise will not generate the same sort of stress as would be the case were the police to arrive on the doorstep to announce he had just been run over by a bus. And this would be particularly true if the poor man had left the house barely a quarter of an hour before to go for a run.

The fatigue that follows bad stress is but the psychosomatic manifestation of "ill-ness" caused by the event. In addition to experiencing a great despondency, which will leave the individual feeling deprived of energy, there may well be symptoms of anguish, anxiety and irritation.

Pathological fatigue

This is dependent on an illness that often has not yet been diagnosed. This is particularly the case with:

- infections: tuberculosis, urinary and pulmonary infection, viral hepatitis

- complications with the endocrine system: diabetes, menopause, hypothyroid, renal malfunction

- metabolic problems: hypoglycaemia, renal malfunction

- circulation problems: pulmonary embolism, low and high blood pressure

- neurological problems: Alzheimer's disease, Parkinson's disease

- inflammatory illnesses

- cancers.

In all these extreme cases, fatigue cannot be overcome unless the treatment for the pathological condition is successful.

Fatigue or tiredness due to poor diet

As already mentioned, the change in eating habits that occurs with some people due to their retirement, health problems or death of their companion, often results in nutritional problems of one sort or the other.

The main nutritional mistakes are the following:

Malnutrition

Either the dietary intake is far too low, or the general dietary level is satisfactory but there is a protein deficiency due to an inadequate consumption of items like meat, fish, eggs and cheese. Both these deficiencies will result in symptoms of fatigue.

It is important to remember at this point that it is possible to be undernourished without being underweight, for the fatty mass and water can be increased at the expense of muscle mass.

Dehydration

In a person weighing 60 kilos (about 132 lbs), a deficiency of 1.2 litres of water in the body leads to a 20% reduction in muscular strength.

And yet an older person, whose awareness of thirst has diminished or even disappeared, will easily reach a deficiency of 1 litre of water in a hot summer, when running a temperature, or when living in an overheated environment.

Micronutrient deficiency

Major deficiencies in mineral salts and trace elements are usually translated into feelings of tiredness. This is particularly the case with vitamins from the B group and particularly vitamins B6 and B9.

However, it is generally the case with all antioxidants: vitamins C and E, betacarotene, polyphenols, selenium, zinc and copper. A deficiency in vitamin D, which encourages osteomalacia or softening of the bones, leads to walking difficulties that can prove exhausting. Also a lack of iron, vitamin C, magnesium and potassium can translate into acute tiredness. Which all goes to show how important it is to have a diet that is nutritionally rich.

Excess weight

Excess weight and particularly obesity can also lead to tiredness and isolation.

Those afflicted are limited in the physical activity open to them. They have difficulty in moving around and often feel soporific.

Hypoglycaemia, a cause of fatigue

The fuel for the body is glucose. The brain, muscles and red blood corpuscles all need it in order to function normally. It is the reason the body arranges for there always to be an adequate level of glucose in the blood - at approximately 1gm per litre of blood.

On awakening with an empty stomach, glycaemia is very close to this level. If we refrained from eating breakfast (something that is not recommended), the body would be able to compensate for several hours, but at the end of the morning, the glycaemic level would be well below what is normal. We could then say that we have hypoglycaemia, with the following symptoms: sudden tiredness, complete exhaustion, sleepiness, irritability, headaches, feeling cold.

After a breakfast consisting mainly of carbohydrates with a high glycaemic index (white bread, sugar, jam, sugared cereals enriched with honey), hypoglycaemia at the end of the morning could be even more pronounced. It is what is called reactive hypoglycaemia, where a *hyper*glycaemia, with an excessive level of sugar in the blood, is transformed into *hypo*glycaemia with a reduced level of sugar in the blood, due to the release of excessive amounts of insulin from the pancreas. In fact, the higher the glycaemia due to the bad carbohydrates, the greater is the risk of forcing the sugar level too low "by reaction". This phenomenon is even more likely after the age of sixty, when there is an increased incidence of hyperinsulinism.

On the other hand, if breakfast is composed of carbohydrates with a low glycaemic index (cereals without sugar, wholemeal bread or bread made with completely unrefined flour, sugar-free jam), the sugar level in the blood rises in a very modest way. As a result, it returns to its normal level in three to four hours, without going through the condition of hypoglycaemia that manifests itself as acute tiredness or fatigue.

It is customary to believe that hypoglycaemia manifests itself with a sudden and marked lowering of the sugar level in the blood, leading to pronounced symptoms associated with fainting: pallor, palpitation, sweating, trembling, acute feelings of hunger and loss of consciousness. Happily, this type of hypoglycaemia is more rare. So-called "functional" hypoglycaemia, which concerns us here, is much more frequent and in all cases where the diet of the patient is modified, these troubles disappear completely.

It has been noticed that certain medications can encourage hypoglycaemia: aspirin, certain antibiotics (tetracylines), haloperidol (neuroleptic), indometacine and betablockers . Hypoglycaemia occurs frequently among unstable diabetics and also among heavy smokers (those that smoke more than twenty cigarettes a day).

Strong coffee and tea, which stimulate the release of insulin, can also encourage hypoglycaemia, as can alcohol - particularly when it is drunk on an empty stomach and when it is combined with sugar (kir, port, muscat, punch, sangria, whisky and coke, vodka and orange).

And then last but by no means least in the impressive list of things that can cause hypoglycaemia, we have stress.

Acidosis

Modern food is very acidifying, something which renders the body more vulnerable to many illnesses and to stress and is often translated into a state of fatigue.

There are acidifying foods and others that are alkalising. It is therefore desirable to find a balance between the two.

ACIDIFYING FOODS	ALKALISING FOODS
Meat, Chicken	Milk
Fish	Yoghurt
Eggs	White cheese
Roquefort, Cantal	Other cheeses
Watercress	Other vegetables
Spinach	Lentils
Sorrel	Haricots beans
Asparagus	Chick peas
Tomatoes	Almonds

ACIDIFYING FOODS	ALKALISING FOODS
Roasted Peanuts	Walnuts, Hazelnuts
Groundnuts	Soya
Sugar, Sweets, Sodas	Wholemeal Bread
Pastries	Bread from unrefined flour
White Bread	Fruit, especially Lemons
Prunes	Dried fruit
Cherries	
Oranges, Grapefruit	
Tea, Coffee, Alcohol	

By way of conclusion, it is important to understand that the lack of performance or energy - or fatigue, to put it more simply - is not a normal state whatever our age, whether we are fifty or twenty-five years old. It is for this reason you do not have to learn to live with it, accepting it as being inseparably linked to the phenomenon of age. The proof of this is that the adolescents of today are often more tired than their parents - even their grandparents. And their perverse dietary fashion, symbolised by hamburgers, chips and coke, is certainly not unrelated.

If it is true that endurance and the power of recuperation are vitiated with age, which is quite normal, the number of years has never justified a chronic state of fatigue. In the majority of cases, the return to a nutritionally rich and varied diet will resolve the problem of fatigue once and for all.

Fatigue foods against performance foods?

We cannot properly speak about foods that lead automatically to states of fatigue, or of others that might allow us to feel supermen within a few minutes after having eaten them. Contrary to what fiction would have us believe, swallowing a tin of spinach, as Popeye did, has never had the same immediate effect as swallowing a potion prepared by the druid Getafix for his friend Asterix.

Fatigue foods

These are rather foods or drinks that should not have been consumed, or should have been consumed with caution so as to avoid the risk of them leading to tiredness:

- taking alcohol on an empty stomach or in excess

- excessive consumption of carbohydrates with a high glycaemic index, which could lead to hypoglycaemia

- eating a meal containing too much fat, which may lead to a long and difficult digestion and to somnolence.

Managing your consumption of wine and fats with care and choosing your carbohydrates judiciously, you can avoid the sudden onset of tiredness in the early afternoon, even after a good lunch in your favourite restaurant.

Performance foods

All foods rich in vitamins, mineral salts and trace elements contribute to a complete and harmonious diet and allow the body to achieve peak performance.

But if you were then to decide to have a meal comprising:

- cod liver for its vitamins A and D

- raw carrots for betacarotene

- kiwi fruit for vitamin C

- wheatgerm oil for its vitamin E

- oysters for their zinc, selenium and copper

- Brewer's yeast for vitamin B

- Gruyere cheese for calcium

- winkles for magnesium

- dried apricots for potassium

- black pudding for iron

- egg yolk for chrome

it is likely you would feel cheated, because apart from the indigestion you would definitely be suffering, it is far from certain you would feel at the peak of your powers. Quite clearly it would not be a nutritionally rich meal that would cause you to jump out of your chair, where you normally take your nap after a meal, straight into the starting blocks for the 110-metre hurdles. However, after two weeks on this energy regime, I am prepared to take a wager that you might!

A more civilised way of achieving the same results would be to arrange your meals over an extended period of time, incorporating the following foods according to your personal preferences:

Breakfast:

Solids:

> Fresh fruit
>
> Wholemeal bread or bread made with unrefined flour
>
> Wholewheat Swedish rolls
>
> Sugar-free cereals
>
> Oat flakes
>
> Sugar-free jam
>
> Yoghurt, 0% fat Fromage Frais
>
> Brewer's yeast, wheatgerm (to add to milk products)

Drinks:

> Low fat chocolate, coffee, tea, chicory, skimmed or semi-skimmed milk, soya milk, freshly squeezed fruit juice

Lunch, dinner:

Solids:

> Crudités (raw vegetables)
>
> Green vegetables
>
> Pulses (lentils, red beans, haricots beans, dried peas)
>
> Fresh fruit

Oleaginous fruit: avocados, walnuts, almonds, hazelnuts

Soya grains and derivatives (tofu, etc.)

Meat, chicken, rabbit, black pudding

Fish, shellfish

Offal (liver, kidneys)

Eggs

Wholemeal bread, bread made with unrefined flour

Brown rice, pasta made with unrefined flour, whole semolina

Cheeses

Chocolate (+70% cocoa solids)

Olive oil, sunflower oil, rapeseed oil

Butter (10 g/j).

However, if on the other hand you prefer a more structured approach, there follows a menu plan for a whole week.

MENU PLAN FOR ONE WEEK

Monday

Breakfast	Lunch	Snack	Dinner
Fresh Lemon juice	Grated carrots with lemon juice	Dried Apricots	Fish soup
1 apple	Salt Pork and lentils	Yoghurt	Brown rice
Wholemeal bread + sugar free jam	Camembert	Tea	Green salad (+olive oil, vinegar)
Yoghurt	Wholemeal bread		Yoghurt
Brewer's yeast	Water		Water
Coffee	1 glass wine		1 glass wine
	2 pieces of chocolate (+70% cocoa)		

Tuesday

Breakfast	Lunch	Snack	Dinner
Fresh Grapefruit juice	Mussels *Marinière*	Fruit according to season	Black pudding
2 kiwi fruit	Salmon with Sorrel	Tea with milk	Celery purée
Wholegrain cereal without sugar	Whole rice		Salad
Fromage frais (20% fat)	Roquefort cheese		Whole semolina cake
Wheatgerm	Bread made with unrefined flour		Water
Coffee	Water		1 glass of wine
	1 glass of wine		
	1 *Espresso* coffee		

MENU PLAN FOR ONE WEEK

Wednesday

Breakfast	Lunch	Snack	Dinner
Fresh Orange juice	Artichoke hearts	Fruit in season	Mushroom omelette
Fruit in season	Guinea fowl	Yoghurt	Chicory salad
Wholewheat Swedish rolls	Stilton cheese		*Crème brûlée*
Yoghurt	Bread made with unrefined flour		Water
Brewer's yeast	Water		1 glass of wine
Coffee	1 glass of wine		
	1 *Espresso* coffee		
	2 lumps of chocolate (+70% cocoa)		

Thursday

Breakfast	Lunch	Snack	Dinner
Fresh Lemon juice	Avocado	Almonds	Fresh tomato soup
Fruit in season	Veal's liver	Hazelnuts	Whole-wheat pasta with basil sauce
Oat flakes	Whole rice	Yoghurt	Salad
Semi-skimmed milk	Cheddar cheese		Yoghurt
Wheatgerm	Wholemeal bread		Water
Coffee	Water		1 glass of wine
	1 glass of wine		
	1 *Espresso* coffee		
	2 lumps of chocolate (70% cocoa)		

MENU PLAN FOR ONE WEEK

Friday

Breakfast	Lunch	Snack	Dinner
Fresh grapefruit	Duck paté	1 hot chocolate drink	Whole semolina
Porridge with semi-skimmed milk	Cod fillet		Ratatouille
	Wholemeal pasta		Salad
Bread made from unrefined flour	Yoghurt		Emmenthal cheese
	Water		Wholemeal bread
Sugar-free Marmalade	1 glass of wine		Water
	1 Filter coffee		1 glass of wine
Tea with milk	2 lumps of chocolate(+70% cocoa)		

Saturday

Breakfast	Lunch	Snack	Dinner
2 kiwi fruit	Crudités (raw vegetables with dips)	Walnuts	Plate of Fruits de Mer (oysters, mussels, prawns, crab and winkles)
Sugar-free wholegrain cereals		Dates	
	Cassoulet (pork and beans)	Tea with milk	
0% fat Fromage Frais + herbs and fresh-ground pepper	Yoghurt		Pancakes
	Wheatgerm		Water
	Water		1 glass of wine
Tea with milk	1 glass of wine		
	1 Espresso coffee		
	2 lumps of chocolate(+70% cocoa)		

MENU PLAN FOR ONE WEEK

Sunday

Breakfast	Lunch	Snack	Dinner
Fresh Orange juice Fruit in season Wholegrain cereal Yoghurt Brewer's yeast Coffee	Roast Beef Cauliflower *gratiné* Ice-cream Jug of cider *Espresso* coffee 2 lumps of chocolate(+70%cocoa)	1 hot chocolate drink	Soya *Galettes* (flat cakes) Carrot and broccoli mousse Mimolette Bread made from unrefined flour Tea

HAVE A HIGH PERFORMANCE BODY

One could say without too much exaggeration that we only use the human body when we do not need it. This is as true of the brain as it is of the muscles.

Be mobile!

Limited physical activity only gives rise to problems, like:

• ankylosis resulting from aggravated osteoarthritis

• breathing difficulties resulting from insufficient use of ventilating muscles

• cardiovascular ailments or diabetes

• aggravation of obesity.

Up to the age of seventy, people are very active. Apart from those who continue to have a professional occupation and the lucky ones who do their garden, there are those who knock things up (in the noble sense of the term), those who travel or those engaged in charity work - without mentioning, of course, those babysitting with the grandchildren! A completely sedentary life is therefore rather rare.

However, that does not prevent certain bad habits developing without our noticing: we take the car to go a few hundred metres and we systematically take the lift, even when we only go to the first floor. Some of us think we should go easy on ourselves by avoiding even the slightest effort, whereas quite the opposite should be the case, for the less we do, the more we accelerate the phenomenon of ageing.

At every age you can swim, cycle or, even better, walk. My grandfather, who lived until he was ninety-one, walked for a couple of hours every day - to go to the office. It is clear that if you want to engage in sport a little more intensively, you should first get the green light from a cardiologist. For those who are too fat, diabetic or merely suffering hypertension, an endurance sport like swimming, cycling or taking long walks, taken under strict medical supervision, can only improve the prognosis for their illness. In fact, it will reduce their hyperinsulinism and insulin resistance.

When we were younger, we did little or no sport, saying we did not have the time. On reaching retirement, we can take advantage of our free time to take up a physical activity again, even if that only means taking walks. We can use the time also to start learning some relaxation techniques, like yoga or meditation, exercises that are particularly good for the highly strung, the emotional and all those who are vulnerable to stress.

All physical activities, including walks, providing they last at least half an hour, improve the rhythm of the heart and blood circulation, control tension and ensure the respiratory muscles maintain their tone. Some retired people retain their youth by taking their grandchildren to and from school. Others use the excuse of having to take the dog for a walk to ensure they get out of the house. If you have no duties of this sort to ensure you keep active, then it is up to you to find some.

Food for exercise

It is a question of knowing how best to feed ourselves before we embark on a serious amount of physical exercise. Many overestimate their powers of endurance when they begin an extended period of exercise - say a hike into the mountains that will result in the body drawing on its reserves of energy over a period of several hours.

It goes without saying that before we get involved in this sort of exercise we should ensure there are no deficiencies in our diet and that we follow the recommendations developed in this book.

Eating before taking exercise

It is important to ensure the body is properly hydrated.

A few hours before we engage in strenuous exercise, we should drink small quantities of liquid at regular intervals. Pure water is best, perhaps laced with lemon juice to prevent acidosis. On no account should we add any sugar, as this could lead to hypoglycaemia during the hours that follow, probably just as we are about to engage in exercise.

The last meal should be taken about three hours before we begin to exercise, choosing carbohydrates with a low glycaemic index. It is advisable to build up as much muscular glycogen as possible, creating a reserve of glucose for the muscles to use when they are working hard.

Lipids and animal protein should be kept to a minimum as they could limit the amount of sugar available to the body by delaying evacuation of the stomach. Too much protein can also aggravate acidosis and increase the levels of uric acid and urea during the course of physical exertion.

So, let us suppose that at 15:00 hours we are going to compete in the senior section of the local cross-country race, here is how we might organise our diet beforehand:

Breakfast at 07:00 hours:

• freshly squeezed lemon juice, with fructose if necessary

• fruit

- wholemeal bread

- stewed fruit, without sugar

- yoghurt

- tea or coffee with powdered skimmed milk

Lunch at 11:30 hours:

- crudités

- wholemeal pasta or past made with unrefined flour, mushroom sauce with a dribble of olive oil

- rice pudding made with skimmed milk and fructose to sweeten

- mineral water

We should eat nothing more after 12:00 hours

Liquids:

- Between 07:30 and 11:30 hours, we should drink unsweetened lemon water, or hot lemon tea if it is cold.

- Between 14:50 and 15:00 hours, we should drink lemon water sweetened with fructose (for 1 litre of water, we need to add the juice of 2 lemons and 60g of fructose). If it is very cold, even add a gram of salt.

Eating during exercise

If our regime has been followed correctly, there will be no risk of hypoglycaemia occurring and if the physical exercise is relatively short (1 hour), there will be no need to drink.

On the other hand, when strenuous physical exercise like skiing, riding, mountain climbing or cycling is prolonged, it is advisable to drink regularly and even to eat. We should prepare two or three litres of the water, lemon and fructose drink described above, and have ready some dried fruit (apricots, figs), wholewheat crackers and bars made from unrefined cereals and fructose.

Nutrition after exercise

If your physical activity has been long and tiring, we will need to recharge your body straight away by eating carbohydrates like chocolate, whole-cereal bars, fresh fruit juice and also potassium in the form of prune juice. We should also drink alkaline water, like Vichy or Badoit, to replace the sodium lost through perspiration.

The next meal should consist of carbohydrates like rice, wholemeal pasta, lentils and dried beans. We should then wait until the following day before having animal protein again.

MAINTAINING SEXUAL VITALITY

Motivation is the name of the game

For a long time, sexuality has been influenced by Judaeo-Christian precepts, according to which the sole purpose of sexual relationships is procreation. As a result, sexual pleasure was condemned. Furthermore, as the subject was taboo, it was not considered good taste to talk about it.

Female sexuality therefore had to repress any eroticism by concentrating exclusively on conjugal duty. As far as the male was concerned, although it was freely admitted he had a more demanding nature, he only managed to satisfy his unnatural impulses after a fashion, thanks to the tolerance of those around him and the hospitality of the oldest profession in the world.

Synonymous with good sense, man's golden age did not easily lend itself to the promptings of sexual desire. Past a certain age, it was more respectable to relegate one's libido to the souvenir cupboard.

For women over sixty, cultural inhibitions are still quite strong in spite of changing attitudes. On the other hand, the pill has helped women before they reach their fifties to disassociate fertility from sexuality. The menopause can therefore interrupt one without calling the other into question. The lack of hormone treatment after the menopause can dissuade active sexuality as the mucous membranes are more dry and fragile. If the vagina is poorly lubricated, coitus is difficult and painful, though this handicap can be overcome with lubricating gels. For a woman on hormone replacement therapy, these problems do not arise and there are other advantages: the skin remains younger, more fine-grained and supple, and ages more slowly.

For men, the male menopause is largely theoretical. In most cases, the secretion of testosterone carries on regardless of age: only the sexual drive diminishes. On the other hand, after the age of seventy-five, statistics show the incidence of dysfunction is more than 50%.

To maintain a healthy sexuality, several factors come into play:

- The need for uninterrupted circulation in the sexual arteries, to ensure erection can occur normally. Any atheromas can obstruct these blood vessels and result in poor erections, leading eventually to impotence. Diabetics are particularly prone to this problem. However, one study has shown that if HDL cholesterol (good cholesterol) is higher than 0.6mg/l, the risk of sexual deficiency is three times less likely to occur than when the level is 0.3mg/l.

- A sound neurological system. Degeneration of the nerves due to diabetes or alcoholism can interfere with an erection.

- Certain medicines promote impotence by causing or aggravating sexual problems. This is particularly true of anti-ulcerative and anticholesterolaemic drugs, betablockers, sedatives and so on.

- On the other hand, a coronary problem is never an obstacle to a normal, healthy sexuality. Just allow yourself to be convinced that the sexual act requires no more effort than that needed to climb two flights of stairs.

- The most important factor is probably the maintenance of regular sexual activity. "Function creates the organ", or at least keeps it in good running condition.

- As with sport, normal sexual relations require regular exercise: otherwise, repeated humiliation in the face of incomplete erections can eventually lead to the abandonment of all endeavour in this area of human activity.

When the physical conditions have been resolved, we can then consider the state of orgasm and libido in the golden age. The work of the famous American sexologists Master and Johnson show that sexual desire and pleasure can still thrive even when sexual relations occur less frequently (on average two to five times a month after the age of fifty). Sexual extinction due to age first comes to those whose sexual lives have never been particularly active.

The real problem exists more at the level of the couple and the harmony to be found there. Does mutual attraction still exist, or has conjugal strife distanced the married couple one from the other?

The remorseless passage of time provides yet another obstacle to male and female libido. The power of seduction may have become a little threadbare. Routine and boredom may have moved in largely unnoticed. In addition to this, the love life of the two partners is rarely synchronised. Just as the woman may have proved unable to preserve her charm and - as common parlance would have it - "has aged badly", it so happens the man is tempted into a clandestine love affair. If an erection proves difficult to realise with a regular partner, the opposite might prove to be the case with another person. Just the novelty factor may prove sufficient to release the log jam. This is what has been noticed in retirement homes, where it is common for new sexual relationships to form even at an advanced age.

Aphrodisiac cooking

We have seen how important it is to have a well-balanced and nutritionally rich diet in order to overcome tiredness and stress. The same also applies to maintaining arteries and nervous system in good condition. Healthy eating makes it possible to avoid the majority of ailments that undermine our sexual vitality.

It is possible on the other hand, to improve our sexual efficiency "naturally" by choosing foods that are reputedly aphrodisiac in their effect.

In the past, sorcerers or old women used to prepare many love potions containing a wide assortment of different substances. Mangadore, a root that vaguely resembled the shape of the human body, was one of the most widely known. According to legend, it was conceived when the sperm of a man being hanged inseminated the earth. Very toxic, mangadore has now disappeared, but many plants with scarcely any symbolism at all have still managed to reach us across the ages. They are used as spices, flavourings, herbal teas or in decoration. Prominent among them are cinnamon, mint, savory, saffron, peppercorn, vanilla, capsicum, nutmeg, clove, coriander, ginger and garlic - exotic flavours you could well consider using in your dishes, as they do in the West Indies.

In addition to spices, some foods have maintained a particular reputation over the centuries for long-known properties that modern science appears to be rediscovering for itself.

Oysters

There is a larger-than-life scene in the film *Tom Jones* where a couple in an inn licentiously devour a large quantity of oysters that have been part of the menu of "bon viveurs" over the centuries. It is said that Alexandre Dumas was capable of eating a hundred or so as an *entrée* to a large meal of many dishes!

Oysters are rich in zinc and it is known that a lack of this trace element can lead to a weak concentration of spermatozoon and weak secretion of male hormones. It is widely known that rhinoceros have been massacred over the years for their horn, renowned in Africa as an aphrodisiac. What is less well known is that it happens to be rich in zinc.

Frogs

The Indian tribes in Brazil still practice a curious custom. The skin secretions of a frog are mixed with saliva and smeared on the chest of the menfolk, who then become drowsy and lie down for about an hour. When they recover, the men are possessed by a very strong sexual urge.

Research workers at the University of Bethesda in the United States have managed to isolate the active substance in these secretions, naming it "adenoreguline" because it works in conjunction with an amino acid called adenosine.

In 1861, Dr Vezien - a military doctor in charge of a field hospital for the Foreign Legion stationed in North Africa - mentioned a strange incident in one of his reports. All the soldiers addicted to eating the legs of the frogs that infested the area, were suddenly afflicted with a priapism - an intense and continued erection normally associated with sexual disease. The doctor administered blood-letting and applied leaches to the affected male members, but concentrated on trying to discover the cause of this curious event. As a result, he observed there were Spanish Flies (Cantharides) in the camp and that they happened to be the favourite food of the frogs in the area.

Now when you crush dried Spanish Flies, you obtain a substance called cantharidine. It is said that this powerful but very toxic aphrodisiac cut short the life of Lucite Borgia and warranted sending the Marquis de Sade to the Bastille for having given rather too much of it to two of his partners in lust - enough, in fact, to poison them.

Recently, the American biologist Thomas Eisner decided to recreate the conditions of 1861 and showed that by feeding Spanish Flies to his frogs and then eating 300g of their legs, there was an indisputable aphrodisiac effect without toxic risk. Bearing in mind what strange things are fed to the animals we eat these days, perhaps we ought to reflect on the experiences of Vezien and Eisner the next time we buy a bag of frozen frog's legs from our local supermarket!

Truffles

If you have decided to break your piggy bank to honour Aphrodite, then go and buy this mushroom that Brillat-Savarin called "the black diamond of the kitchen". He went on to add: "It awakens erotic and gourmand memories in both sexes, for it makes women more tender and men more enterprising."

Our modern pharmacologists have shown that truffles contain a vegetable hormone, androstenone, similar to the male hormone testosterone. This explains why they used to hunt truffles with a sow on heat, because she could smell minute quantities of this substance even when the mushroom was buried several inches below the surface of the earth. The molecule is also present in the pheromones of human sweat, which encourage sexual excitation and apparently 92% of women are affected by it.

Fresh truffle is certainly more expensive, but it contains double the amount of androstenone present in preserved truffle. And in matters of love, we should never count the cost!

Celery

In antiquity, this fragrant plant was used in the crowns prepared to honour the virile and valorous conquerors in the games at the circus.

In the twelfth century, the abbess St Hildegarde mentions it in her treatise on medicine, "in order to stimulate creative ardour". A popular proverb used to say: "If a woman knew what celery does for a man, she would travel from Paris to Rome to find it."

Recent chemical analyses have shown that wild celery (or apium) - and only that variety - contains androstenone and alkaloids that stimulate the contraction of the muscles of the perineum. So it really is a food to arouse physical desire.

Chocolate

The aphrodisiac qualities of chocolate have been known since the time of the Aztecs. To honour the women in his harem, King Moctezuma was happy to drink forty cups of it a day. However, it should be said that during this period, chocolate also contained many spices, like chilli, cinnamon and cloves, all of which were well known for their aphrodisiac properties.

To be more certain her lovers would come up to expectations and before letting them into her bed, Madame de Pompadour would make them drink two cups of chocolate with triple vanilla. As far as Casanova was concerned, he often gave thanks for this "beverage of the gods" (theobroma cacao), for helping him cope with the bulimia of female conquest to which he was so prone.

In fact, cocoa contains tonic substances such as caffeine, theophylline, theobromine and even an antidepressant, phenylethylamine. Moreover, when we eat chocolate, the feeling of pleasure causes the secretion of endomorphines in our body - morphine produced internally that gives us a feeling of well-being.

So even if chocolate (bitter chocolate contains at least 72% cocoa) cannot be properly called an aphrodisiac, it does at least put us in the mood and makes us feel happy. What better prelude could there be then, for the act of love?

Champagne

This is the only aphrodisiac "food" manufactured by man. In small quantities - that is to say, a couple of flutes - it removes inhibitions and promotes desire. So says Dr Tran Ky. Madame Pompadour, unquestionably an expert on love, said this about it: "It is the only wine a woman can drink, without becoming ugly."

However, it must be consumed in moderation, as too much alcohol kills love and gets in the way of sexual performance. For as the proverb says: "Bacchus is the enemy of Venus".

But beyond the more-or-less theoretical effect of these foods, let us admit that the best aphrodisiac for a man will always be the desirable woman.

MENU SUGGESTIONS FOR A ROMANTIC MEAL

———

Hot oysters cooked in Champagne
Frog's legs with garlic and savory
Boar with fresh truffles and purée of celery
Chocolate gateau laced with ginger
Champagne

———

A meal created by Bartolomeo Scappi, cook to pope Pius V
"prepared in 1568 for a gentleman happy with life....":

Amourettes (bull's testicles),
cooked in pepper, nutmeg, oregano,
thyme and garlic

———

A menu proposed by her doctor Nicolas Venette,
for Madame Pompadour:

Celery soup
Truffles
Hot chocolate with ambergris and vanilla

———

An experimental menu recommended by Oscar Wilde in 1890:

Cancale Oysters
Foie gras with truffles from the Périgord
Partridge with paprika.

FOODS THAT ACTIVATE SEXUALITY

Oysters	Frogs	Celery	Tomatoes
Truffles	Chocolate	Verbena	Ginger
Champagne (no more than 2-3 flutes per day)			Saffron
Garlic	Peppers	Rosemary	Cloves
Cinnamon	Vanilla	Peppercorn	Savory
Nutmeg			

Avoid lettuce and tobacco.

STRENGTHENING THE BRAIN TO IMPROVE YOUR MEMORY

The brain deteriorates with lack of use

In the absence of much cerebral activity, the neurons of the brain disappear more quickly than would normally be the case. Conversely, if there is significant activity going on, involving important intellectual work, then the natural ageing process of the brain is slowed down.

Many people who have lost the habit of using their memory are able to describe actions and events that occurred in the Second World War, but are unable to tell you what happened the previous week and even less where they put down their spectacles ten minutes before. Their recollection of the past is almost intact but their recollection of today's events is less than fresh. They complain about their memory but never about their laziness! However, maintaining a good memory is principally a question of willpower.

Although he was seventy-eight years old at the end of his second seven-year term as president, and was suffering with cancer, François Mitterand was still able to dazzle negotiators and staff with his excellent memory.

Every three months there used to be a big reception at the Elysée Palace, during which he would present a dozen or so *Légions d'honneur*. On these occasions, the President would give a speech to each recipient lasting ten minutes, when he would refer to the professional achievements - with supporting dates - that had made them worthy of receiving such high national distinction. Without exception, all those attending these events - including his political opponents - could not help but admire and be amazed that François Mitterand could make his twelve speeches without ever referring to a note.

Even if you are never able to be as impressive as this, because it takes many years of training, you can still improve your memory significantly. What is more, it is never too late to start. Many books have been published recently, giving wise counsel on exercises to apply and how to train. But as always, the food you eat can not only help you keep your memory but also improve it.

Diet and cerebral ageing

Several nutritional mistakes help to speed up cerebral ageing and undermine our intellectual faculties:

- a general reduction in energy intake, particularly protein intake

- a low intake of polyunsaturated fats, which build up the phospholipids in the membrane of cerebral neurons

- a lack of antioxidants to protect phospholipids from the peroxidation of free radicals

- a lack of glucose, the sole energy source for brain cells, caused by an unbalanced diet or by hypoglycaemia, will change the way the brain works. This underlies the importance of eating carbohydrates with a low glycaemic index, which will help maintain stable sugar levels in the blood during the course of the day.

In view of their wealth of important nutrients, Brewer's yeast and wheatgerm are indispensable additions to your daily diet.

On the other hand, aluminium figures prominently among the poisons that can undermine the functioning of the brain and it should never be allowed to come into contact with your food. Aluminium utensils and aluminium foil should therefore be excluded permanently from the kitchen.

Deficiency in	Consequences and Symptoms	Foods to overcome the deficiency
Vitamin B1	Memory problems Irritability Tiredness Depression Lack of appetite	Brewer's yeast Wheatgerm Peanuts Pork Offal Unrefined cereals
Vitamin B2	Memory problems Tiredness Character problems Nausea Low blood pressure	Brewer's yeast Eggs Mushrooms Meat Unrefined cereals Pulses
Vitamin B6	Memory problems Tiredness Abnormal irritability Depression Anaemia Sugar craving	Brewer's yeast Wheatgerm Soya beans Offal Meat Fish Brown rice
Vitamin B9	Lapses of memory Tiredness Mental confusion Depression	Beer yeast Dried beans Wheatgerm Animal liver Oysters
Vitamin B12	Memory problems Sleeping problems Irritability Depression Difficulty in walking	Animal liver Kidneys Heart Herring Mackerel Rabbit Oysters Fish

Deficiency in	Consequences and Symptoms	Foods to overcome the deficiency
Magnesium	Reduced vigilance Reduced intellectual faculties Susceptibility to stress	Winkles Wheatbran Wheatgerm Cocoa powder Pulses Nuts Unrefined cereals
Phosphorus	Losses of memory Reduced vigilance Somnolence Modified taste	Brewer's yeast Cheese Soya bean Chocolate (cocoa 70%+) Fish

Alzheimer's disease

This is a disease much talked about these days and it is important to mention it here because it is affecting more and more elderly people.

Quite obviously attempts have been made to see whether there are any nutritional causes and several theories have been put forward, listing possible causes such as:

- a lack of vitamins A, B1, B6, B9, B12, C, D and E

- disruption of the enzymes involved in the fight against free radicals

- a lack of iron

- the toxic effects of aluminium

- an excess of zinc

- a lack of glucose in certain regions of the brain.

However, none of these theories have been supported formally and, without doubt, the illness is caused by several factors. This is why it has been suggested likely causes could be immune problems, a virus, abnormalities in neurotransmitters. So far, no line of enquiry has resulted in an effective treatment being discovered.

FOODS GOOD FOR THE MEMORY

Brewer's yeast, wheatgerm

Unrefined cereals without sugar

Cocoa powder

Chocolate (containing more than 70% cocoa)

Tea

Fresh fruit

Oleaginous fruit: walnuts, almonds

Soya beans

Mushrooms

Green vegetables

Seaweed

Pulses: lentils, haricot beans, peas, broad beans

Winkles

Oysters

Fish

Liver, kidneys

Eggs

Meat

Ginger

Clove

Take an interest in everything

Two factors that are complementary and indivisible play a key role in holding back the ageing process:

• The nutritional factor, which is the concern of the main part of this book.

• The psychological factor, or the state of mind in which we find ourselves.

I had the good luck to live several years with my grandmother, who lived until she was 102 years old. Everybody who knew her will recognise her from the brief description that follows.

She was the personification of *joie de vivre* and had a particularly well-developed sense of humour. Always happy, full of fun and entertaining, for her life was a permanent farce in which she laughed as much at herself as she happened to laugh at others.

Her concern with her personal appearance was legendary. From the moment she got up to the moment she went to bed, she was immaculate - dressed, coiffured and made up as if she were a duchess at the Court of Versailles. "You", said the postman who liked to tease her, "you could be invited to a wedding at the very last minute, because you are always ready." She had such a young air about her that when the doctor asked her for her age, she would quite happily knock off a quarter of a century without anyone thinking of taking her to task. When she was already over a hundred years old, a touch of bronchitis kept her in bed for a few days. On that occasion she was treated at home. However, by the second day she had asked for the young nurse to be replaced because she had refused to apply her make-up for her.

Born in 1882, she was therefore eighteen years old in 1900. She had witnessed the introduction of electricity, the telephone, the motor car, the aeroplane, radio and television. Technological progress fascinated her and her dream was not only to fly on Concorde but also to travel to the moon. I never heard her say "Oh, things were better in my day!", because she always lived in the present and was always making plans for the future. Even at the age of ninety-six she was planning her holidays for the following year.

She listened a lot to the radio. Politics was her favourite subject. Every day she read the newspaper and when she acquired a television, she never missed the current affairs programmes. Her knowledge of national and international events was impressive and she loved to engage in discussion with anybody prepared to listen, though the conversation soon became light-hearted.

For her, eating was always an event. Even when she was completely on her own, the table was set as for a banquet. Besides champagne - she always looked for an excuse to open a bottle - she only drank red wine at the table (a Bordeaux more than five years old) and would remind everyone as if in justification, that "if Jesus used it as a symbol of his blood, then it must be good for your health". She would not dream of missing Christmas Eve. Even when she was a hundred years old, I saw her have her oysters and foie gras at two o'clock in the morning, then - totally at ease with the world - go to bed at five, after having opened all her presents.

When we look around at people of my grandmother's age, there are some like her, but they are rather rare. We are more likely to see sad people - people locked up inside themselves, harping on about the past, without hope, without desire and without plans for the future. How can we expect such people to enjoy a party on Christmas Eve, or New Year's Eve for that matter?

Loneliness is often the result of a state of mind. If we are happy and open to the world, if we are interested in other people, then they will come to us. We complain too often about being lonely, when we should complain about the way we shut ourselves in: for if we want to be accepted, then we have to accept the world around us first.

For those who have retired and want to come out of their shell, there are more than enough opportunities to do something. First of all, we can make ourselves useful, because real happiness comes with giving. We can help children, family, friends or neighbours, and the personal satisfaction that comes as a result far outweighs the small amount of effort required on our part. Or we can participate in group activities, whether local, secular or religious. Many of those who have given a little of their time to those less fortunate that themselves have discovered a new meaning to their lives. Then there are all those activities that not only help us use our time intelligently but bring us into contact with lots of other people: gymnastic clubs, bridge clubs, dancing classes, university courses for the retired, cultural trips and so on.

If you have to single out a fundamental rule, then it is this: make certain you are fully occupied. Structure your activities, have a diary to organise all those events and opportunities that never fail to crop up. When the system is up and running, see to it that you are so busy you scarcely know which way to turn in order to cope. Selfishness, being wrapped up in yourself and inactivity, are the great precursors of pessimism, boredom and loneliness.

When you were the slave of your job, you always complained you never had time to go to the cinema or the theatre, to read books, travel, do odd jobs, garden or engage in sport. However, from now on you are totally free to pursue all your hobbies. So make the most of it.

To find out how you are shaping up, I am going to suggest that - right here in the middle of this book - you do the following: take a fresh piece of paper and answer these questions: What did you do yesterday, hour by hour? What are your plans for tomorrow? For the coming months?

If there is not much to report or if what you have listed bores you, then go on to list your interests and perhaps even go on to list the chores that laziness has made you postpone.

Sort out some objectives and do some planning. You will see that if you have due regard for life, it will never cease to fascinate. This is because, as with professional life, retirement must be active!

The elderly can find themselves in three different scenarios that require a different nutritional response:

- Perhaps there is no particular health problem, but in the past the family appears to have been susceptible to certain illnesses we would prefer to avoid. This worry is understandable. However, if we have arrived at the age of seventy without mishap, it is not very likely we will suddenly succumb to an hereditary disease; it would have manifested itself long since.

- Or perhaps there is a minor health problem that requires a specific diet to prevent the condition becoming worse.

- Or then again, maybe there is a serious health problem that has given rise to a heart attack for example, and everything must be done to avoid there being a recurrence.

This is exactly what we shall be examining in the chapters that follow when we look at what we need to do "when the engine starts to misfire".

2 Learn how to manage your weight

For several decades, excess body weight has been a major problem in Western society. Today, the criteria for being considered slim have become more and more rigorous - firstly for medical reasons, where it has been shown that excess weight is a risk factor as far as health is concerned, but mainly for aesthetic reasons. As a result, all methods for losing weight are of interest to the general public at large and the media have not been slow in profiting from this interest: at regular intervals they inundate their readers with semi-sensational articles that have no purpose other than sell paper and perpetuate our dreams.

There are many widely held ideas regarding diets, and if it is already dangerous to do anything and everything to lose weight when we are young, then it is particularly dangerous to do so when we are in our fifties. This chapter should therefore help you get your bearings on the subject.

Variation in the components of body mass

What is not generally realised when we step onto our bathroom scales is that they will only give us our overall weight. And this, of course, is only part of the story.

The other part of the story is that with age, the fatty mass and water in our bodies increase at the expense of lean mass: this means that having a so-called "normal" bodyshape and weight are not necessarily factors that guarantee we have a healthy, well-nourished body.

Only impedancemetrics make it possible to calculate the percentage of water, lean mass (muscles) and fatty mass in the body. The body mass index (BMI - see formula on page 204) and the height/hip ratio give a clearer idea of the proportion of fatty mass and its distribution in the body.

Corpulence after fifty

A number of studies conducted on people over sixty have allowed us to appreciate their average BMI and to draw some general conclusions:

- 45% of men and 55% of women have a BMI higher than normal

- among these, 20% of men and 30% of women are sufficiently overweight to warrant a loss of weight

- average corpulence of those studied, remains constant with age and even has a tendency to diminish over time.

What is an ideal weight?

It is probably healthy to lose a few kilos at the age of fifty, but a person over seventy with a limited amount of extra weight does not have a problem. Such a condition could even be considered an advantage, as these energy reserves will prevent such a person becoming undernourished in the event of illness.

This means the idea of being overweight needs to be adjusted as a function of age. A BMI of 28 is too high for a person when they are fifty years old, but quite acceptable when they are seventy. However, before we go on to discover what we can do about losing weight without endangering our health, let us first examine various types of obesity.

Classification of obesity

We can identify three types of obesity:

Android obesity

It is found mainly on the upper body: the face, neck, chest and abdomen above the navel. Men with bellies bulging above their belts are good examples of this type. The condition manifests itself after fifty years of age and more frequently with men than with women.

In case of doubt, android obesity can be determined by taking a tape measure and checking the chest measurement/hip measurement ratio. The condition is deemed to exist when the ratio is less than 1 in the case of men and less that 0.85 in the case of women.

Gynecoid obesity

This condition mainly affects women and manifests itself before the age of fifty. Fat is deposited principally in the lower part of the body, in the lower abdomen (below the navel), as well as on the hips, thighs and buttocks.

Metabolic effects are rare, but they are often accompanied by venous insufficiency giving rise to varicose veins and, about the age of fifty, a painful osteoarthritis in the lumbar region of the spine, in the hips and in the knees. However, the main harm is in fact, aesthetic.

A complication of this type of obesity is usually cellulitis, with which it is often confused. Gynecoid obesity is a diffused fatty infiltration of the body cells, whereas cellulitis is made up of localised fatty deposits, trapped and encapsulated in fibrous tissue.

Deep abdominal obesity

This is the most difficult form of obesity to diagnose and is the most dangerous. It exists in people who have a normal corpulence and are not overweight. However, it is a genuine obesity in that the fatty mass is significant though not apparent. It is generally discovered by chance during surgery on the abdomen or when the patient is being scanned for a minor problem like lumbago.

It is present as a very widely spread fatty mass deep in the abdominal cavity, enveloping all the organs. Prognosis is poor because it can quickly prove fatal following the onset of metabolic complications.

Is it necessary to slim?

Trying to lose weight beyond a certain age can be tricky because we need to know whether such a step is justified. We must therefore weigh the pros and cons.

In the case of a man

• Up to the age of sixty-five, losing weight is justified in order to avoid heart attacks.

• From sixty-five to seventy, slimming may be justified if there is a precise medical condition that requires it - for example, a coronary attack associated with high cholesterol levels or diabetes.

- Beyond the age of seventy, losing weight is not desirable unless excess weight is contributing to mechanical problems - difficulties with walking, or osteoarthritis occurring in the hips or knees. However, the existence of metabolic problems does not justify losing weight unless the patient is seriously obese (with a BMI above 35).

In the case of a woman

- Before the age of fifty, the risks associated with being overweight are mainly linked to venous problems and osteoarthritis.

- Around the age of fifty, managing the menopause becomes a priority, though contrary to popular belief, it does not necessarily lead to wait gain.

- After the age of fifty, in the absence of hormone treatment, cardiovascular risk can be a problem, particularly for those suffering with android obesity. For those suffering with gynecoid obesity, there are no medical risks - the only harm is aesthetic. As far as women receiving hormone treatment are concerned, there is no inherent vascular risk, though slimming might be justified if diabetes is present.

Medical risks associated with diabetes

Obesity may be responsible for the following metabolic complications that often accompany it:

- hyperinsulinism with insulin resistance

- diabetes type II (non insulin dependent)

- hypercholesterolaemia, with the risk of coronary attacks

- hypertriglyceridaemia

- hyperuricaemia.

Respiratory problems

But there can be problems on the respiratory front. The obese can in fact suffer with ventilatory problems that restrict the amount of air finding its way into the lungs. The most frequent problem is sleep apnoea (respiratory arrest lasting at least ten seconds and occurring more than five times an hour). Only a partner is likely to notice this interruption to the breathing cycle, which will normally accompany bouts of snoring. Apart from the danger of the breathing cycle being permanently interrupted in severe cases, the patient may suffer with bouts of abnormal sleepiness during the day, headaches, memory problems and so on.

Rheumatological problems

Excess weight displaces the centre of gravity of the body. With the tummy projecting forward, certain mechanical stresses in the joints appear:

• pains in the back

• tendonitis in the knee

• osteoarthritis of the hips and knees.

In addition, there is a greater sensitivity to pain leading to an increase in the incidence of rheumatological pain.

Cancer and obesity

With men, obesity brings an increased risk of cancer occurring in the prostate, colon and rectum. In the case of women, there is an increased risk of cancer occurring in the uterus, breast, ovaries and gall bladder. However, the overweight who need reassurance should bear in mind that thin people (with a BMI under 23) run the greater risk of contracting cancer.

Surgical risk

Cardiac and respiratory disorders and the increased risk associated with phlebitis, all add to the risk the obese undergoes on the operating table. The healing of wounds is often delayed and skin infections are more frequent.

Psychosocial repercussions

Being overweight is generally more widely accepted among the elderly than among the young, even if aesthetic worries still persist.

Nevertheless, repeated attempts to lose weight by following severe diets have often resulted in the obese being marginalised, which can cause them to develop psychological disorders such as anxiety, depression and food cravings.

The effects of weight loss

Reducing body weight by 5 to 6 kilos is sometimes sufficient to bring high blood pressure back to normal, even if ideally the subject should shed a further 10 kilos. It is important an elderly person should not be too zealous in trying to achieve their goal weight but should be content with a partial result. It is far better to lose just a third of your excess weight rather than lose more initially to put it on again later, as it has been shown statistically that fluctuations in body weight (the so-called "yo-yo" effect) contribute substantially to cardiovascular risk.

Because of this risk, many nutritionists often advise patients not to diet if they are only marginally overweight.

Can obesity be beneficial?

This question may appear preposterous. However, we can ask ourselves whether excess weight may not have certain benefits. Statistics show in fact, that men over sixty have less risk of dying if their BMI lies between 26 and 28 - that is to say, on the verge of being overweight.

In particular, the risk of dying of cancer is clearly higher if you are slim (with a BMI lower than 23) as opposed to fat (with a BMI over 28).

With women over fifty and after the menopause, being overweight helps guard against osteoporosis, as part of the excess fat changes into hormones that prevent the reduction of bone mass.

Does the menopause make you fat?

Comprehensive statistics on the weight of French women as they progress from the age of twenty to the age of fifty-two show there is an average increase of 10 kilos, from 54 to 64 kilos.

We are often inclined to believe that the menopause is one of the main factors responsible for this increase in weight. However, when we plot the curve for weight gain over the years, we find there is a very marked slow-down in the rate of increase from the age of forty-five.

In fact, if we examine the statistics closely, we notice two things: only 43% of women have a problem with putting on weight at the time of the menopause (4 to 6 kilos) and weight gain is much lower when a woman is having hormone treatment (31%).

Moreover, the experience of doctors shows us that women who put on weight at the menopause (with or without treatment) are always those who happen to be overweight already.

All of which leads us to think that, contrary to some widely held views, the menopause is not a determining factor in weight gain but rather an amplifying factor. If a woman has a strong tendency to become fat, it is probable she will put on additional weight during the menopause.

The best way for a woman to avoid doing this is for her to modify her dietary habits. This is, in fact, what the Montignac Method suggests and what I would invite you to discover in the next chapter.

3 The Montignac Method: a simple dietary adjustment

In nature, corpulence and obesity, its extreme form, do not exist. No trace of it can be found among wild animals and in primitive societies it is rarely recorded.

On the other hand, the phenomenon is less exceptional in great civilisations, but each time it is observed, it is always in very specific socio-professional groups:

- Roman patricians or certain military commanders when the empire was collapsing

- certain ecclesiastics, particularly monks

- some aristocrats, but above all the bourgeoisie of the post-industrial revolution.

In every case, they were individuals belonging to favoured groups. This is why it was long thought that being "robust" was solely the privilege of the rich. Thus it was inferred that corpulence was the result of a diet that only the rich could afford.

This idea is quite wrong. Today, in industrialised countries, we see it is particularly among the poor that we find the most obese people.

For many years, the phenomenon of excess weight went largely unnoticed and it was even thought to be a sign of good health. And then in the middle of the twentieth century, the situation began to change, starting with the United States.

It was noticed there that the average weight of Americans was beginning to increase in an alarming manner and that contrary to what had been believed, corpulence constituted a health risk. Scientists at the time therefore formulated a theory: if the inhabitants of rich countries were becoming fatter and fatter, it was because they were eating too much and exercising too little. The human body, they thought, functioned like a boiler. To live, it needed energy from food.

There was thus an energy input on the one hand and an output on the other. Corpulence leading to obesity, was therefore the result of an imbalance between inputs and outputs of energy expressed in calories.

This is the hypothesis on which the theory of the low-calorie diet has been constructed. From this was born conventional dietary practice, based on a voluntary restrictive approach having the following two principles:

• eat less by counting calories

• spend more time doing a lot of exercise.

Today we have experimental proof that this hypothesis is wrong. To understand why this is so, we must first refer to some facts and observe particularly what has happened in the United States.

Here is a country which, for more than forty years, has stubbornly applied these two principles with great determination. As a result 65% of all Americans are overweight and 20% of them are obese. What is more, we know this situation has worsened considerably since this restrictive dietetic came into widespread use. A part of the scientific community that has quite rightly denounced this scandal has stated categorically: "The main cause of obesity is the systematic following of successive low-calorie diets."

It is a view supported by the statistics. Contrary to what has been believed, only 15% of those who are obese eat more than average. On the other hand, 30% eat normally and 50% far less - often very little.

Here is a paradox we can understand if we reflect a little. Each time a living being is frustrated, it develops a reactionary behaviour. If undernourished, its instinct for survival will cause it to organise itself so that it can build up reserves. An organism subjected to dietary restrictions will therefore change its energy output: it will start to use less energy in order to keep more in reserve. So paradoxically, when we restrict our food intake, we accomplish the opposite of what we are trying to achieve because the less we eat, the fatter we become.

Scientific studies have proved that contrary to what was originally thought, the human body does not function like a boiler. We now know it is not the energy content of our food or the lack of energy expenditure in physical exercise that explains corpulence. So what does?

WHY DO WE BECOME FAT?

We will discover that it is actually the nature of the food we eat - its nutritional content – that is indirectly responsible for us becoming fat. It is the nutritional characteristic of our food that will - or will not – promote the metabolic processes leading eventually to weight gain.

To understand the processes underlying the formation of fat reserves, we must first unearth some very simple technical ideas.

Glycaemia

Like everybody else, you will certainly have had your blood analysed at some time. Among other things, your doctor will have checked the level of your glycaemia - that is to say, he will have checked to see whether the quantity of sugar present in your blood is more or less than normal (1g per litre of blood).

The presence of sugar - or more exactly, of glucose - is important, because it is the fuel of the body that replenishes itself continuously from body reserves. When the glucose level (which acts as a sort of gauge) descends well below 1g per litre, the body is then said to be in a state of hypoglycaemia. At this point the pancreas will secrete a hormone, glucagon, which will immediately convert glycogen (a body starch stored in the muscles or liver) or even body fat, into glucose.

When the glucose level in the blood goes beyond 1g per litre, then the body is said to be in a state of hyperglycaemia. On an empty stomach, this could indicate a prediabetic condition and be the reason for the doctor requesting a blood test. However, hyperglycaemia is otherwise a normal condition that results from eating carbohydrates (often loosely termed sugars) in the form of cereals like wheat and maize, starchy foods like dried beans, lentils and potatoes, or again fruit. When we eat a carbohydrate, the metabolic process it undergoes in our body will automatically give rise to hyperglycaemia.

As it would be dangerous for the body to remain in this condition, the pancreas - yet again! - secretes another hormone, insulin, to bring blood sugar levels down to normal by storing excess glucose in the body for future use.

For a long time, scientists thought the glycaemic potential of carbohydrates was uniform. This is why the consumption of carbohydrates by diabetics was restricted indiscriminately. Then, in 1976, Professor Crapo, an American authority on diabetes, discovered that blood sugar levels generated by carbohydrates could vary considerably from one to the other. In the case of potatoes, white flour and sugar, the level was very high; but in the case of fruit, lentils and dried beans, it was low. He therefore had the idea of classifying carbohydrates according to their glycaemic potential and then called this classification the Glycaemic Index.

Hyperinsulinism

When we eat a carbohydrate like bread, we have seen how there is a rise in our blood sugar level that prompts the pancreas to respond by secreting insulin to bring the level down to normal. When the pancreas is in good condition, the amount of insulin secreted is proportional to the level of glucose in the blood. However, when the pancreas is working badly, it will secrete more insulin than is required to reduce glycaemia to normal levels. This excessive secretion is called hyperinsulinism.

Now we have known for several years, as a result of scientific studies, that hyperinsulinism is the real cause of weight gain. In fact, it has been possible to show that excessive secretion of insulin will cause the fatty acids circulating in our blood after our last meal to be stored abnormally in our body as fat reserves.

To understand this phenomenon properly, we will study an example. Martin has a strong tendency to put on weight. Bearing in mind what we have just said, it is reasonable to assume that his pancreas is not in a very good condition and that he is suffering from hyperinsulinism. We will give him two apparently identical consecutive meals and observe what happens.

In the first meal, he will be served a nice pork chop representing 600 calories and potatoes cooked in the oven representing a further 400 calories. A total of 1,000 calories.

In the second meal, Martin will be served salt pork with lentils. The knuckle of pork will represent 600 calories and the cooked lentils served with a trickle of olive oil, will add a further 400 calories.

The two meals are apparently identical. Their composition in terms of proteins, lipids and carbohydrates are more or less the same, as is their energy content of 1,000 calories.

Let us see then, what happens at the metabolic level. In the first meal, the potatoes with a high glycaemic index of 95 will lead to an important increase in blood sugar levels. Martin's pancreas will therefore secrete a large amount of insulin, but as it is in poor condition, it will secrete more than is required. It is precisely this excess of insulin (hyperinsulinism) that will cause the major part of fatty acids circulating in the blood, from the pork fat eaten during the meal, to be stored in the body. Martin will therefore put on weight.

In the second meal, as the lentils have a very low glycaemic index of 30, the concentration of glucose they will generate in the blood will be very weak. The corresponding secretion of insulin will therefore be modest, insignificant. In any event, certainly not enough to induce the slightest hyperinsulinism. In this case, none of the fatty acids circulating in the blood will be stored as body fat. Martin will therefore not put on weight!

These two scenarios not only help us understand the metabolic mechanism that causes us to put on weight, but also show us that, contrary to what some nutritionists wrongly maintain, the energy component in food is not the determining factor in weight gain. For in these two examples, Martin absorbs the same number of calories in each meal, the same energy content in meat, particularly in fats, and the same energy content in starches. And yet, in the first meal he puts on weight and in the second he does not.

The Glycaemic Index

So what is it that makes Martin put on weight when he eats one meal as opposed to the other?

The answer lies in the nature of the starch - in its nutritional content, particularly as indicated by its glycaemic index. The higher the glycaemic index of the food eaten, the more it will give rise to hyperinsulinism that will trap the fats eaten during the same meal.

When this phenomenon has been properly understood, it is easy to see that becoming overweight, then corpulent and finally obese, is only the result of the type of food we choose to eat. If we mainly eat foods with a low glycaemic index, like unrefined cereals (wheat, oats, unrefined flour), legumes (dried beans, lentils, broad beans), fruit and the majority of green vegetables, we do not run the risk of getting fat, however much energy we absorb from other foods like meat, fish, eggs, cheese and oils. This, incidentally, is the way our ancestors used to eat.

On the other hand, if we largely confine ourselves to eating foods with a high glycaemic index, such as refined flours and their derivatives (white bread, white pastas, pizzas, cakes, biscuits, crackers), sugar, potatoes or white rice (which is also refined), then we must not be surprised if we get fat. As we have seen earlier, fats eaten during the same meal will be trapped and stored in the body by hyperinsulinism for which the pancreas will become increasingly responsible.

Unfortunately, this way of eating is widespread in industrialised countries. Choosing the wrong foods really does lie at the heart of weight gain and we will see later what we should do to normalise the situation.

First it is important to discover why there has been such a major shift in the dietary habits of modern society during the last two centuries and particularly during the last forty years.

Let us begin by looking at the glycaemic index table overleaf. This classification is a scale of values based on the arbitrary value of 100 given to pure glucose. In the left-hand column we have listed all the foods with a glycaemic index over 50. In the right-hand column, we have listed all those below this value.

When we look at the column of carbohydrates with a high glycaemic index, there are two things we should notice.

As expected, sugar features in the list with a GI of 75. However, we also see listed, mashed potatoes or, even worse, roast potatoes (with a GI of 95 when a raw potato only has a GI of 70). It was a Frenchman called Barnes who showed that the way a food was cooked could increase the glycaemic potential of a food. We see this to be the case not only with the potato but also with maize. Cornflakes and popcorn have a GI of 85, whereas maize in its natural state has a GI of 70.

The second thing to note is that the foods in the column on the left, with a GI over 50, are modern foods - foods that have become popular in recent decades. Three in particular now used excessively in Western diets, scarcely existed at the beginning of the nineteenth century. These are sugar, refined flour and the potato.

Sugar

Before the sixteenth century, sugar was practically unknown in the Western world. Sometimes it was used as a spice, whose rarity made it very expensive,

GLYCAEMIC INDEX OF VARIOUS CARBOHYDRATE FOODS

Carbohydrates with a high Glycaemic Index		Carbohydrates with a low Glycaemic Index	
Maltose (beer)	110	Wholemeal bread; bran bread	50
Glucose	100	Brown rice (Western)	50
Potatoes (roasted or fried)	95	Garden peas	50
Very white bread	95	Breakfast cereals, unrefined,	
Mashed potatoes	90	unsweetened	50
Parsnips	90	Spaghetti (Durum), *al dente*	45
Honey	90	White rice, sticky (Oriental)	45
Carrots, cooked	85	Oats (lightly rolled)	40
Corn flakes; popcorn	85	Kidney beans	40
Rice, easy cook	85	Fresh fruit juice, unsweetened	40
Broad beans, cooked	80	Pastas made from	
Swedes	80	unrefined flour	40
Pumpkin	75	Pumpernickel (black, rye bread)	40
Watermelon	75	Rye bread, unrefined	40
Sugar (saccharose)	70	Bread, unrefined flour	35
White bread (French Baguette)	70	Dried peas	35
Breakfast cereals, sweetened	70	Dairy products	35
Chocolate bars	70	Ice Cream (lightly sweetened)	35
Potatoes, boiled	70	Carrots, raw	30
Biscuits	70	Dried beans	30
Modern maize/corn on the cob	70	Lentils	30
Noodles, Tagliatelle	70	Chick peas	30
White rice (Western)	70	Pastas made from	
Brown Bread	65	unrefined flour	30
Dried fruit	65	Other fresh fruits	30
Potatoes cooked in their skins	65	Jam made without	
Beetroot	65	sugar/grape juice	30
Bananas; melons	60	Black chocolate (> 70% cocoa)	22
Jam made with sugar/grape juice	60	Fructose	20
Spaghetti (Durum), well cooked	55	Soya	15
		Peanuts	15
		Fresh green vegetables	15
		Mushrooms	15

attainable only by the wealthiest. The discovery of the New World made a limited development of sugar cane possible, but transport and the cost of refining always ensured it remained a luxury product reserved for the privileged. In 1780, consumption was less than one kilo per inhabitant per year.

However, the discovery in 1812 that sugar could be extracted from beet gradually turned sugar into a major consumer product with an ever-decreasing cost price.

Since then, the annual consumption of sugar per head of the population in the Western world has increased dramatically. The statistics for France are as follows:

1800	0.6 kilo
1880	8 kilos
1900	17 kilos
1930	30 kilos
1990	35 kilos

- though it should be borne in mind that the French eat less sugar than any other group in the Western world. The English, for instance, currently eat 50 kilos, the Germans 54 and the Americans 63!

The increased availability of sugar has completely transformed the dietary habits of our contemporaries. We could even say that never in the course of human history has there been so radical a change in the diet of mankind within such a short space of time and with such far-reaching consequences. For, due to its high glycaemic index, sugar gives rise to hyperglycaemia and excessive stimulation of the pancreas.

Flour

As far as flour is concerned, the process of bolting has always taken place. This process, which involves passing the flour through a sieve to separate it from the bran, used to be done by hand. However, bearing in mind the costs involved (30% of the flour was eliminated in this way), bolted flour was reserved for the privileged few.

As ordinary people only had the right to eat black bread - not bolted, that is! - one of the main demands of the French Revolution was white bread. However, it was necessary to wait until 1870 and the invention of the roller mill before the cost of bolting was reduced sufficiently to produce refined flour at a realistic price.

Partially refined initially, black bread only became white after the First World War and very white (hyper-refined) more recently. However, it is important to realise that the refining process can produce flour with a glycaemic index that will vary between 35 and 85, reaching GI values that will cause blood sugar levels to soar. Refining flour will also remove most of its nutritional content (fibre, vitamins, mineral salts, trace elements, proteins, etc.), leaving starch, which is only of relative interest.

With the exception of the Americans, we probably eat less bread than we did a century ago but far more white flour.

Potatoes

In view of the vast quantities eaten, we might be forgiven for thinking that potatoes belong to the dietary heritage of old Europe. In fact, this is not the case, as it only began to be part of our staple diet during the course of the eighteenth century after it was used as a replacement for wheat during the famines that preceded the French Revolution.

Since its discovery in Peru in the middle of the sixteenth century, the potato had only been used to fatten pigs. It was even called the pig tuber and such was the suspicion in which it was held, because it belonged to a botanical family where most of its species are poisonous, that eating it was even forbidden by the Church.

However, what interests us today is to discover that the potato has one of the highest glycaemic indexes - higher even than that of sugar - and its nutritional content is so poor, its store of vitamins, mineral salts and trace elements are all located on the outer layer of the skin. As a result, what little nutrition is contained in a potato is systematically removed when they are peeled!

Dietary habits

When we look at the table of carbohydrates classified according to their glycaemic index, we cannot help but be struck by the fact that the majority of the foods on the right, like unrefined cereals, legumes (lentils, dried beans, peas, broad beans) and all the green vegetables, are mainly those that were eaten in former times, whereas those on the left are foods we prefer to eat today. From this we can conclude that over the last one hundred and fifty years - and particularly over the last forty years - there has been a pronounced change in dietary habits that has led us to forgo a low glycaemic diet in favour of a high glycaemic one. Statistics confirm this: for example, these days the French eat eight times fewer legumes than they did fifty years ago.

So it is this dietary change that has progressively raised the average blood sugar levels of our fellow citizens, producing the chain reaction which is now all too familiar: hyperglycaemia, leading to hyperinsulinism, leading to the storage of fatty acids.

This study of the glycaemic index table of carbohydrate foods, also allows us to understand better why the United States has an incidence of obesity that is far higher than that in France: it is clearly because the American diet is made up almost exclusively of foods coming from the bad index column. Judge for yourself:

Americans eat:

• sugar (63 kilos per person per year)

• foods containing white or super-white flour: sandwiches, hot-dogs, hamburgers, pizzas, pastas, cookies, crackers

• potatoes (even for breakfast!)

• maize or sweetcorn (principally in the form of popcorn and cornflakes, both of which have a very high glycaemic index).

In the main, Americans eat foods that raise their blood sugar levels and lead to hyperinsulinism. As they eat a lot of meat - together with its fat - they stockpile the risks of storing the corresponding fatty acids as fat reserves.

An additional reason why Americans have a higher incidence of obesity than we do is quite simply that they changed their dietary habits before we did.

In point of fact, three factors are involved in the process of putting on weight.

• The first is the diet factor - food that raises blood sugar levels and overstimulates the pancreas with the dire results already alluded to.

- The second is the time factor - to give rise to hyperinsulinism, the pancreas must be over stimulated for an extended period of time. This accounts for the fact that slim people who are careless about the food they eat because they are slim can eventually develop a weight problem.

- The third is the individual factor - some people are more fragile, more sensitive than others. Their pancreas is destabilised more rapidly. Alternatively, they may have an inherited predisposition. If their parents are fat, there is a likely predisposition to hyperinsulinism and very soon they may show signs of obesity.

And then, at critical moments in their lives - and this is particularly true of women - the body may be more vulnerable when the hormone balance in the body is disrupted, either during adolescence, pregnancy or the menopause. However, in all these scenarios, it is always bad dietary habits that trigger or aggravate the condition.

When casting a final eye over the table of glycaemic indexes, some will not fail to be astonished at the fact that rice has a high index despite the fact it is the staple food of Asiatic people who do not suffer from obesity.

The explanation is simple: Asiatic rice, which is by definition "sticky", contains an important amount of soluble fibre that lowers its glycaemic index. The opposite is true of "gluey" Western rice. What is more, Asians, who use rice as a source of energy, always eat it with lots of vegetables that are high in fibre and have a very low glycaemic index. As a result, their meal has a very low overall glycaemic index.

Similarly with the poor of yesteryear, whose diet was based on the potato eaten with lots of vegetables or legumes that helped reduce the overall glycaemic index of their meal to acceptable levels.

The tragedy of our modern diet is that with the rise in our standard of living, we replace vegetables with meat whilst keeping rice and potatoes as an accompaniment. In this way we combine the two elements that lead to weight gain: foods with a high glycaemic index and fats.

For a long time, people have been mystified by the fact that maize, with its apparently high glycaemic index, was for centuries the staple diet of the American Indian. But the explanation is simple. Modern maize is a hybrid plant selected by agricultural scientists for its high yield, whereas traditional Indian maize was much harder, more coloured and contained more soluble fibre (and essential nutrients), which ensured it had a low glycaemic index.

The modern variety, on the other hand, is nutritionally impoverished and has a higher glycaemic index.

In fact, all modern cereals selected for their yield rather than their nutritional properties, have a higher glycaemic index than the varieties cultivated in the past. A return to the cultivation of those ancient varieties would therefore seem to be a natural, beneficial and obvious step for us to take today.

So, by a simple reorientation of our dietary habits, consciously choosing to eat foods with a low glycaemic index, we can resolve the problem of being overweight. This is the message that lies at the heart of the Montignac Method.

THE MAIN PRINCIPALS OF THE MONTIGNAC METHOD

The Montignac Method is simple because it is based on making the right choice of foods. This is the reason we can say that it is selective but, unlike low-calorie diets, never restrictive.

In fact, it is convivial, because it can be followed wherever we are - either in the home or in the restaurant, entertaining friends or associates. It is even gastronomic, inasmuch as it allows us to enjoy our food and eat foods that are the basis of classical cuisine.

The Montignac Method unfolds in two phases, even though the first is not really necessary for those who only have a few kilos to lose.

Phase I

This is the weight-loss phase which lasts, from one to three months and is the time it takes to change our dietary habits: giving up the bad and choosing the good - choosing "good" carbohydrates and "good" fats. It is a time when we allow the body to recover its equilibrium - a time when we will make little or no demands on certain metabolic functions - like pancreatic secretion, for instance.

It is a phase that is easy to cope with because it imposes no restrictions in term of quantity of food that may be eaten. For those who hold low-calorie diet season tickets, we might say this phase is even a pleasure because they can at last slim and eat at the same time!

On the other hand, Phase I is selective, in the sense that certain foods are excluded - such as "bad" carbohydrates - or eaten in a certain way at one particular moment during the day. It is easy to apply, particularly in those cases where meals have to be taken outside the home. Meals will be varied and the diet balanced, rich in protein, fibre, vitamins, mineral salts and trace elements.

Generally speaking, this phase does not give rise to feelings of frustration, for those able to eat their fill, experience feelings of intense satisfaction when each day they notice the benefits brought by this new dietary method.

Its guiding principle is the rotation of protein-carbohydrate and protein-fat meals for breakfast, lunch and dinner, whilst making sure the carbohydrates eaten are always those with a low glycaemic index.

Depending on the number of kilos to be lost, Phase I can last between two to three months.

EXAMPLES OF MEALS (PHASE I)

Protein-Carbohydrate (without fats)

Breakfast	Lunch	Dinner
Orange	Grated carrots	Cucumber with fat-free yoghurt dressing
Wholemeal Bread	Lemon juice	
Jam (sugar or grape juice free)	Brown rice	Lentils with tomato sauce
Decaffeinated tea or coffee	Soya sauce	
	Raspberries with fructose	Cooked prunes
Skimmed milk	Water	Water

Protein-Fat (without carbohydrates)

Breakfast	Lunch	Dinner
Scrambled eggs	Smoked salmon	Curly endive with
Bacon/ham	Grilled steak	lardons
Decaffeinated tea or	French beans	Poached cod
coffee	Cheese	Broccoli
Semi-skimmed milk	Water	Cheese

EXAMPLES OF MEALS (PHASE II)

Breakfast	Lunch	Dinner
Apple	Grated carrots with	Mushrooms *à la*
Wholemeal bread with	olive oil vinaigrette	*grecque*
butter	Roast leg of lamb	Wholewheat pasta and
Jam (sugar or grape	Dwarf kidney beans	tomato sauce
juice free)	Cheese	Parmesan cheese with
Tea/Coffee	Wine	olive oil
Semi-skimmed milk		Walnuts
Mandarine	Oysters	Leeks vinaigrette
Muesli	Calf's liver	Haricot beans with
Jam (sugar or grape	Broccoli	walnut oil
juice free)	Cream caramel	Mozzarella cheese
Semi-skimmed milk	sweetened with	coated with cream
	fructose	Wine
		Coffee/tea
Orange juice	Foie Gras	Avocados with shrimps
Porridge	Toasted wholemeal	Lentils with olive oil
Full cream milk	bread	Full-fat yoghurt
Hazelnuts or almonds	Smoked salmon	Wine
Coffee/Tea	Parsley mushrooms	
	Chocolate mousse	

Phase II

This phase is a natural extension of Phase I and should be considered as a relaxed cruising phase that will last indefinitely - a sort of gastronomic holiday that will, in a year or two, become a way of life.

We should never forget that eating carbohydrates with a low glycaemic index is a fundamental element of the Montignac Method. However, as time goes by and we become more familiar with the method, we can afford to be more relaxed about the carbohydrates we eat. We can indulge our whim for the occasional roast potato (cooked with goose fat, of course!) or the occasional pastry, but we must never lose sight of the fact that these whimsical forays do our bodies no favours and we should compensate accordingly – either by increasing our fibre intake to lower the average glycaemic index of the offending dish or by going back to Phase I for our next meal.

General recommendations for Phase I

- Only eat wholemeal bread or better still, bread made from unrefined flour

  With a protein-carbohydrate breakfast: no limits.

  With lunch and dinner: only occasionally if you must, to accompany foie gras or cheese.

- Eat raw food as much as possible:

  Crudités

  Smoked or marinated raw salmon

  Steak Tartare.

- Cook at low temperature or in a steamer as much as possible, and do not overcook.

- To avoid possible digestive problems, only eat raw fruit at breakfast on an empty stomach or between meals. Fruit eaten at the end of a meal should be cooked.

- Eliminate all carbohydrates with a high glycaemic index, in particular:

  Sugar (replace with fructose)

  Potatoes (replace with lentils, beans, peas)

  Refined white flour (in white bread, pastas, cakes)

  White, "gluey" Western rice. White "sticky" oriental rice is acceptable, providing it is steamed or eaten together with the liquid in which it was cooked.

  Maize or sweetcorn.

- Do not drink more than one or two glasses of liquid per meal.
- Never drink alcohol on an empty stomach. Always eat something beforehand.

(For more information on the Montignac Method, you may wish to refer to *Eat Yourself Slim....and Stay Slim* published in 1999.)

4 Reduce the risk of cardiovascular disease

Heart disease is still the main cause of death in France despite the fact that the incidence has declined and cancer is always on the increase.

CAUSES OF DEATH IN FRANCE

Types of disease	1980	1991	Rate of Change
Not differentiated	547,000	524,000	- 4%
Cardiovascular	204,400	175,000	-14%
Cancer	128,600	143,200	+12%

However, when we talk of cardiovascular disease, we need to distinguish between:

- Coronary disease - angina pectoris (angina) and myocardial infarction (restriction or complete blockage of one or more the coronary arteries to the heart).

- Problems associated with cardiac rhythm - tachycardia (abnormally high heartbeat), bradycardia (abnormally low heartbeat) and arrhythmia (irregularity or loss of heart rhythm).

- Blood pressure - the pressure exerted by blood against the arterial walls, which decreases with distance from the heart. It is considered to be abnormal if the systolic pressure, when the heart contracts, is above 160 mm or if the diastolic pressure, when the heart dilates, is above 115mm.

- Cerebral haemorrhage or stroke, caused by a crack developing in a blood vessel in the brain due to excessive blood pressure.

- Cerebral thrombosis or ischemic stroke, caused by the formation of a blood clot in a vessel supplying blood to the brain.

• Arteritis (inflammation) of the peripheral arteries, which corresponds to the progressive obstruction of the arteries in the lower body.

An atheroma consists of a fatty deposit on the wall of a blood vessel. Like fur in domestic plumbing, atheromata reduce the diameter of the blood vessels and if the blood is too thick, they will allow blood clots to form. Should they become dislodged and travel round the body in the blood, they will eventually come to rest and obstruct the arteries (coronary, pulmonary or cerebral).

Death as a result of coronary heart disease remains an important factor after middle age, causing the demise of 76% of men over the age of sixty-five and 83% of women over the age of seventy-five. However, it should be pointed out that these medical "accidents" come at the end of a pathological process spread over several decades.

Quite clearly it is important we should do our best to prevent a cardiovascular problem from developing, by putting in place a healthy lifestyle as soon as possible and adopting a minimum of nutritional precautions. Medical studies have shown, in theory at least, that from the moment of pregnancy we should start to give the child a diet that will give protection against cardiovascular disease. Be that as it may, it is never too late to be aware and to act.

THE FACTORS RESPONSIBLE FOR CARDIOVASCULAR DISEASE

If we want to take preventative measures, it is a question of knowing on which parameters we are going to act. For some time through the popular press, there has been a tendency to ascribe to cholesterol much of the responsibility for cardiovascular disease. This has obscured other risk factors that, over the years, have emerged as important in the development of the disease. Besides, several factors acting together can increase the global risk and have a much more catastrophic effect on the prognosis of the disease than we might imagine.

Cholesterol

Even if it is unfair to charge it with all the faults, it has been shown that with increased levels of cholesterol there is a greater risk of death resulting from a coronary heart attack.

However, it has been noticed that for the same average cholesterol level the incidence of coronary illness will vary from one country to another. This would seem to indicate that there are other factors involved in the equation that need to be studied.

For example, in Ireland where they have an average cholesterol level similar to that in France (2.2g/l as opposed to 2.25g/l), deaths from coronary disease are about 5.5 per 1,000, whereas in France it is only 1.4 per thousand (figures include all age groups). Also, a large study undertaken for the World Health Organisation has shown that in France, the mortality rate is three times lower than in the United States where the average cholesterol level is slightly lower than in France.

The discovery of these important differences with their attendant commentaries gave rise to the famous "French Paradox", which explains them in terms of dietary differences between France and the United States.

Bearing in mind the number of risk factors that exist, the above findings show it is not very reasonable to lower cholesterol levels without regard to the consequences. In fact, if this obsession with reducing cholesterol levels is pursued too rigorously, the results can even be dangerous. For example, if the level of cholesterol in the blood falls below 1.7g/l, other risk factors begin to appear: nervous depression, violent death, suicide and increased incidences of cancer. In fact there is a correlation between excessively low levels of cholesterol and cancer, though it is not possible to say which factor determines the other.

As we have seen previously, it is the relationship between "good" (HDL) and "bad" LDL cholesterol that matters. Dietary counter-measures will therefore address this worry by increasing the amount of good HDL cholesterol eaten and decreasing the amount of bad LDL.

We must remember that someone who is very much overweight can bring down high blood cholesterol and even blood pressure to normal levels, merely by losing part of their excess weight. Putting a healthy diet in place is therefore the first step to take, well before prescribing medication.

Unfortunately, general practitioners who received little formal training in nutrition when they were students, are rather prone to "prescribe medication" - a course of action permanently encouraged by the pharmaceutical industry.

Professor Apfelbaum, who courageously and scientifically attacked our current "anti-cholesterol" obsession, has excited the wrath of fellow doctors unable to accept his advice that they should leave well alone and not prescribe diets and medication to people who were not in fact ill. These "patients" suddenly appeared in the statistics at the end of the eighties, when the Americans decreed new and much stricter standards for blood cholesterol levels. As a result, from one day to the next, millions of Americans who thought they were not at any risk, found themselves labelled "ill" and the consumption of medication for lowering cholesterol increased by a factor of ten!

And all this was done for the greater happiness of the pharmaceutical industry that undoubtedly originated this move, which was amply supported by warnings from scientists with impeccable credentials duly appointed by those same pharmaceutical laboratories.

Triglycerides

For a long time it was believed that a high triglyceride level (TGL) in the blood (over 1.5g/l) was only harmful if it was associated with high levels of cholesterol. However, a few years ago it was shown that too many triglycerides on their own constituted a fully-fledged cardiovascular risk.

A study has shown that the risk of a coronary heart attack is increased:

• by 30% if the TGL is above 1.4g/l

• by 65% if the TGL lies between 2 and 4g/l

• By 340% if the TGL is above 4g/l.

Although triglycerides are lipids, it is rarely the case that too high an incidence in the blood can be blamed on food intake, but rather:

• Either too much sweet food - in which case it will be necessary to eliminate visible sugar in the form of lumps, grains, sweets and jams, and invisible sugar in the guise of biscuits and pastries.

• Or too much alcohol. A high TGL in this case is not necessarily due to alcoholism, but rather hypersensitivity to alcohol. Even an intake of less than 30g per day can give rise to excessive levels of triglycerides. The cause can be due to:

Medication

Oestrogens (pills, treatment for menopause and some betablockers)

Some diuretics

Cortisone

Retinoids

Obesity   In this case, weight loss is sufficient to reduce TGL

Fat diabetes.

So, what do we have to do to lower triglyceride levels?

- In the case of diabetics and the obese, it will be sufficient to lose weight.

- If there is no weight problem, however, then we must first eliminate all alcoholic drinks for a period of ten days. If the triglyceride level reduces to normal, we have the proof that alcohol was the cause of the problem. If it does not, then we must eliminate all sweet foods and carbohydrates with a high glycaemic index (white flour, baked potatoes or chips).

- In all cases we should eat fish - preferably fatty fish like salmon, mackerel, sardine and tuna - as it is the only food that will actively improve our TGL: 30g of fish per week should be sufficient to obtain satisfactory results.

Hyperglycaemia and hyperinsulinism

These are two ailments that affect diabetics and the obese, and which also affects the elderly fairly frequently. We know they favour vascular lesions and, as hyperinsulinism generally develops into insulin resistance, there is, in addition, a hardening of the vascular walls and a thickening of the blood that can lead to the formation of clots blocking the arteries.

Any treatment that does not aim to correct hyperinsulinism, will allow the risk of cardiovascular complications to continue by default.

There are two effective solutions to correct matters: one is to take sufficient physical exercise (in agreement with the cardiologist) and adopt a diet that is based principally on the consumption of low glycaemic index carbohydrates - cereals without sugar, unrefined foods (pastas, bread, rice), dried vegetables, fruit and green vegetables.

Hyperuricaemia

The walls of the arteries are likely to deteriorate if the level of uric acid in the blood is allowed to exceed 70mg/l and it should be remembered that there is a greater incidence of myocardial infarction among people suffering with gout. But we will deal more fully with this problem in chapter 6.

The lack of antioxidants

As we have already seen, free radicals are widely implicated in cardiovascular attacks and diabetes. We know they indirectly contribute to the death of cells and bring about what amounts to the rotting and rusting of our bodies.

It is important therefore, that our diet should supply sufficient antioxidants in the form of vitamins A, C, E, selenium, zinc, copper and polyphenols. As it has not yet been shown that food supplements containing these substances are effective, it is preferable to ensure that our daily diet contains enough of these antioxidants to meet our needs.

A healthy lifestyle

In addition to organic causes, certain additional factors can directly or indirectly favour cardiovascular diseases.

Tobacco addiction

At the level of cardiovascular disease, the effects of tobacco are well known. Essentially they are due to the harmful effect of nicotine, which brings about:

• An increase in blood pressure

• An increase in "bad" LDL cholesterol

• A decrease in "good" HDL cholesterol

• A reduction in vascular cross-section due to atheroma

• An increase in the viscosity of blood - the most important cause of thrombosis

• A reduction in the oxygenation of body tissue.

Moreover, because the smoker has a profoundly altered sense of taste and smell, there is a tendency to eat too much fat (particularly saturated fat), which brings out the aroma of foods, and salt. Furthermore, cigarettes rob the smoker of a vast amount of vitamin C, aggravating the deficit existing in this area.

Stress

Two types of sufferers have been identified. Type A, who is very tense, moves constantly not knowing when to stop to breathe, is constantly overwhelmed by excessive hyperactivity. Type B, who is a worrier, anxious, not very outgoing and keeps thing close to the chest.

Type A is the one who is most exposed to cardiovascular risk. Type B is more likely to develop stomach ulcers, colitis and all other sorts of psychosomatic symptoms.

Physical inactivity

A lack of physical exercise is an aggravating factor as far as cardiovascular risk is concerned. But without necessarily engaging intensively in a sporting activity, daily life offers all sorts of opportunities to stir ourselves: walking, taking the stairs instead of the lift, etc.

DIETARY PREVENTION OF CARDIOVASCULAR DISEASE

Basically this will involve selecting specific macro and micronutrients, according to the metabolic effects they will have on the cardiovascular system.

Choice of fats

It is quite possible to cook delicious meals without using fats:

• Meat can be grilled or tossed in a non-stick frying pan

• Fish can be poached in a court-bouillon, steamed or cooked in tin-foil

• As far as vegetables are concerned, they are best steamed. It is the best cooking method for saving most of the micronutrients.

CHOICE OF FATS

Foods to avoid	Foods for limited consumption	Foods for normal consumption	Foods to be encouraged
Margarine	Fat meats	Lean meat	Fatty fish
Suet	Delicatessen meats	Lean delicatessen meats	(salmon,
Lard	Offal	Eggs	mackerel,
Palm oil	Chicken skin	Poultry	sardine, tuna)
Crème fraîche	Viennese pastries	Semi-skimmed milk products	Rapeseed oil
Cooked butter	Biscuits	Cheese	Natural Yoghurt
Paraffin oil	Pastries	Foie Gras	Sunflower oil
Full cream milk products	Butter (10g/day)	Goose fat	Wheatgerm oil
		Duck fat	Corn oil
		Walnuts	Olive oil
		Oleaginous fruit	
		Black chocolate (+70%)	

FATS FOR COOKING

To avoid	To use
Butter	Olive oil
Lard	Goose fat
Margarines	
Palm oil	
Hydrogenated fats	

Choice of proteins

Distinguishing between proteins in terms of the role they may play in cardiovascular illness is still an area that is largely unexplored. However, we do know that fish protein is preferable to protein from ordinary meat and delicatessen meat.

What is more, vegetable protein is preferable to animal protein: for this reason, we should think in terms of eating soya and all its by-products, as well as legumes (lentils, dried beans, peas....) and unrefined foods.

Some of the protein in milk could consititute a risk factor. However, this problem disappears if the dairy product is fermented. Even when made from full-fat milk, certain strains of bacillus in yoghurt can cause cholesterol levels to go down, and it has been clearly shown by the MONICA study that there is no correlation between the importance of eating cheese and the frequency of cardiovascular disease.

Choice of carbohydrates

As we have already said, we have to select foods with a low glycaemic index: sugar-free unrefined cereals, wholemeal bread or bread made with unrefined flour, wild or unrefined rice, pastas made with unrefined flour, lentils, dried beans, fresh fruit, oleaginous fruit, green vegetables.

It is a choice that has the advantage of providing vegetable protein, fibre and a good intake of micronutrients. However, it also helps to correct hyperinsulinism by keeping blood sugar levels low.

Eat plenty of fibre

This requirement is fulfilled when we choose to eat carbohydrates with a low glycaemic index.

The effect of fruit rich in pectin - a soluble fibre - is particularly clear. Different studies have shown that by eating three apples a day:

• Blood sugar levels are lowered were they a little too high in the first place

• Cholesterol levels above 2.8 g/l are reduced by 5%

• Bad cholesterol (LDL) is reduced by 13%

• Triglycerides are reduced by 5 to 10%

By increasing the amount of pectin eaten still further, cholesterol and triglyceride levels can be reduced by more than 20%.

Eat foods rich in antioxidants (see page 51 for list)

Here is how we could construct a menu that would give us a good intake of antioxidants during the course of a day:

Breakfast

   Lemon juice

   2 kiwis

   Wholemeal bread or bread made with unrefined flour + butter

   Semi-skimmed chocolate milk

Lunch

   Oysters

   Calf's liver + broccoli and lentils

   Yoghurt + Brewer's yeast

   Glass of wine

Snack

   Hazelnuts, almonds

   Fresh or dried apricots

   Green tea

Dinner

Grated raw carrots and red cabbage with *fines herbes* and olive oil

Salmon and wild rice

Watercress salad dressed with walnut oil

Roquefort cheese

A glass of wine

Other foods to keep an eye on

Potassium

Taken in sufficient quantities, potassium protects against blood pressure and cerebrovascular attacks.

It is found particularly in the following foods:

• Brewer's yeast

• Dried apricots

• Lentils

• Haricot beans

• Split peas

• Prunes, dates

• Almonds, hazelnuts, walnuts

• Mushrooms

• Black chocolate (+70% cocoa solids).

Magnesium

A diet lacking in magnesium can give rise to high levels of triglycerides in the blood, increase "bad" cholesterol (LDL) and decrease "good" cholesterol (HDL). It has been known for a long time that the incidence of deaths due to heart attacks was higher in those regions where tap water was poor in magnesium.

Moreover, magnesium has been used with success in the emergency treatment of myocardial infarction. It also helps keep blood pressure under control, perhaps due to its regulatory effect on the nervous system and because it reinforces tolerance to stress.

It is to be found particularly in the following foods:

• Winkles

• Wheatbran

• Cocoa powder

• Wheatgerm

• Soya beans

• Almonds

• Brewer's yeast

• Haricot beans

• Bread made with unrefined flour

• Lentils.

Calcium

It probably has a beneficial effect in the fight against blood pressure.

Sodium

To combat high blood pressure, it has long been the practice to prescribe a low-salt diet. We now know this treatment is not always effective: many young adults, for instance, are insensitive to a diet without salt. With elderly people, however, this is less often the case.

Contrary to what we might have expected, a diet very low in salt (below 1 gram per day) will increase cholesterol and therefore cardiovascular risk.

Iron

Oxygen-greedy iron is suspected of aiding and abetting the action of free radicals. This is why we should not blindly supplement our diet with iron.

Vitamin B9 (folic acid)

Many studies have shown that a lack of vitamin B9 contribute to cerebrovascular accidents that are unfortunately fairly frequent in the case of the elderly and which frequently result in paralysis.

Drinks

Drink Wine

Too much alcohol undeniably contributes to the formation of triglycerides, as well as giving rise to arterial lesions and blood pressure.

All the beneficial properties of wine we are about to describe occur only if consumption is moderate and on a regular daily basis - that is, 20 to 30 grams of alcohol per day, or two to three wine glasses. If consumption is sporadic, say only at weekends, then the results are quite different.

With a regular intake of wine as described, we will notice the following:

• An increase in "good" (HDL) cholesterol

• A lower aggregation of plaques, due to a more fluid blood forming fewer clots

• A strengthening of the vascular walls

• An antioxidant effect brought about by polyphenols

• A correction of insulin resistance.

Recently, even small doses of aspirin have been found in wine - an interesting discovery, because aspirin has been used in therapy for a long time as a preventative measure against cardiovascular attack.

This protective effect is practically non-existent with beer, and in the case of spirits (distilled alcohol produced by chemical synthesis), the effect is quite the reverse, as they aggravate vascular risk.

Coffee

For a long time coffee was blamed for contributing to cardiovascular disease. In reality, the statistics were flawed because big coffee drinkers are also smokers.

When all other parameters - particularly nicotine addiction - are removed from the statistics, coffee does not have a harmful effect, except when it is boiled. The practice of boiling coffee, which still persists in some regions of France (in the North, for example), causes a 5 to 10% increase in LDL cholesterol.

With people sensitive to caffeine, coffee (not decaffeinated) can aggravate hyperinsulinism, particularly in the case of the obese and Type II diabetics.

Tea

Green tea only infused for a short time, is poor in theine (identical to caffeine) and rich in polyphenols. As a result, it has an interesting role to play in cardiovascular prevention. However, we should not overindulge nor over infuse, as an excess of tannin stimulates the absorption of iron.

However, black tea - as widely drunk in France - appears to have no particular properties.

Chocolate

Cocoa butter contains fatty acids that have a beneficial effect on cholesterol levels. Black chocolate is also very rich in fibre (14g per 100g of chocolate containing 84% cocoa solids).

As a drink at breakfast time, we could use a cocoa with a low sugar content, similar to the type produced by *Van Houten*. On the other hand, we should avoid milk chocolate (saturated fatty acids) and chocolate containing a lot of sugar (likely to cause hyperinsulinism).

Milk

Drinking full-fat milk is not advisable for those with cardiovascular problems. Skimmed milk is normally recommended for its important calcium content, although, as we have already seen, a large number of the elderly have difficulty digesting it. In which case, it can be replaced with soya milk enriched with calcium.

Sugared drinks

They should be avoided, bearing in mind the risk of hyperinsulinism they pose. Instead, drink squeezed fruit juice (particularly from lemons, as they alkalinise the blood, which reduces the vulnerability of the body to stress).

The power of condiments

Basil

Basil is rich in potassium, calcium, magnesium and vitamin C. It therefore helps prevent the onset of cardiovascular disease and reduces blood pressure.

Garlic

The beneficial effects of garlic in relation to cardiovascular disease are well known. It inhibits the formation of plaques in the arteries, thereby improving blood flow and avoiding the formation of blood clots. In addition, it reduces the levels of sugar, triglycerides and LDL cholesterol in the blood, without affecting the level of "good" HDL cholesterol.

A study of 432 people suffering with cardiac insufficiency has shown that the half of the group that had the juice of garlic added to their drink each day over a period of three years had a mortality rate twice as low as the control group.

THE MEDITERRANEAN DIET

As we saw from the table at the beginning of this chapter, despite having a diet that is more "fatty" and a cholesterol level that is higher, the French in general - but particularly the French in the Mediterranean area - suffer less from coronary disease than either the Americans or the Irish.

We talk about a "French Paradox", but when we look at the figures, we can see that although France may not be a large country, there are big regional disparities because eating habits vary considerably between one province and the other.

In the north, they prefer to eat meat, potatoes, chips, butter and beer. In the south, they prefer fish, pulses, raw vegetables, garlic, olive oil and wine. Now, every year there are 30% more heart attacks in Lille (a city in northeast France) than there are in Toulouse (in the south).

With regard to cooking, in Lille 80.6% use butter and 10.2% use lard (both saturated fats). In Marseille, not far from Toulouse, 65.1% cook with olive oil. During the survey, 75% of the people interviewed in Lille said they ate a lot of delicatessen meats: in Marseille this percentage fell to 49.5%.

In the Mediterranean area, Crete has the lowest incidence of cardiovascular disease. So, what do the Cretans eat? Their diet is rich in mono-unsaturated fatty acids (olive oil), fish, bread made from coarsely bolted flour, pulses, onions, garlic, basil and other herbs, all washed down with wine. It is characterised by a large intake of fruit and raw vegetables as part of a structured meal. There are no snacks between meals.

As a result, we have a diet that is rich in antioxidants, essential fatty acids, oleic acid and fibre. Statistically, it is the importance of eating fruit, raw vegetables, olive oil and wine that is the principal element behind the "French Paradox" and the effectiveness the "Mediterranean diet" in preventing cardiovascular disease.

There are two types of disease prevention: primary prevention, which hopes to delay the onset of illness thanks to a well-balanced diet, and secondary prevention, which occurs if a specific diet prevents the recurrence of a medical accident that has already taken place.

When prescribing a Mediterranean type of diet, Professor Renaud noted a 75% reduction in the recidivity of myocardial infarction in patients under the age of seventy who had already had a heart attack. In this group, only 1% of patients died through infarction and 1% through cerebral vascular accident, as opposed to 5.5% and 6% respectively in the control group.

The recommended Mediterranean diet therefore includes:

• Little meat - preferably chicken

• Fish, twice or three times a week

• Bread (preferably made with unrefined flour)

• Pasta and rice (preferably unrefined)

• Pulses: lentils, chick peas, kidney beans

• Crudités: raw carrots, cabbage, onion, tomatoes, lettuce

- Green vegetables: peppers, courgettes, French beans, broccoli

- Condiments: garlic, basil, parsley, onion

- Olive oil - but also rapeseed oil, and walnut oil

- Very small amounts of butter; no cream or margarine

- Cheese, at least once a day

- At least one fruit a day

- Two or three glasses of wine daily.

PREVENTION OF CARDIOVASCULAR DISEASE

Highly beneficial foods
Olive Oil
Fish
Walnut oil
Duck and goose fat
Wine
Foie Gras
Garlic
Apples (fruit)
Dark chocolate (+70% Cocoa solids)
Wheatgerm

Fairly beneficial foods
Sunflower oil
Rape seed oil
Raw carrots
Horseradish
All types of crudités
All green vegetables
All pulses (lentils, dried beans,
peas, chick peas)
Avocado
All fresh fruit
Oysters
Yoghurt
Oleaginous foods

Neutral foods
Poultry
Rabbit
Game
Eggs
Shellfish

Unrefined cereals
Rice (except sticky)
Fermented cheese
Skimmed milk products

Risk foods
Meat
Delicatessen meats
Offal
Semi-skimmed milk products
Goat's cheese
Cakes and pastry
Viennese pastry
Biscuits
Spirits
Sugar
White flour
Sticky rice
Baked or fried potatoes

High-risk foods
Fatty meat
Fatty delicatessen meats
Butter
Crème fraîche
Full milk
Bacon
Lard
Margarine
Palm oil
Copra oil

PREVENTION OF CARDIOVASCULAR DISEASE WEEKLY MENU

MONDAY

Breakfast	Lunch	Teatime	Dinner
Freshly squeezed lemon juice Fruit in season 1 yoghurt Oat bran Chocolate + skimmed milk	Crudités with vinaigrette Tuna Unrefined rice Cheese Wholemeal bread Water Glass of wine Espresso coffee + segment of dark chocolate (+70%) *(Optional)*	Green tea Walnut	Vegetable soup Unrefined pasta, with trickle of olive oil Salad Yoghurt Water Glass of wine

TUESDAY

Breakfast	Lunch	Teatime	Dinner
Freshly squeezed orange juice Fruit in season Wholemeal bread + sugar-free jam 1 yoghurt Wheatgerm Coffee	Tomato salad Rabbit and Mustard sauce Fresh wholemeal pasta *Oeufs à la neige* (with skimmed milk) Water Glass of wine Espresso coffee + segment of dark chocolate (+70%) *(Optional)*	Green tea Fruit in season	French onion soup Scrambled eggs Salad Cheese Wholemeal bread Water Glass of wine

PREVENTION OF CARDIOVASCULAR DISEASE WEEKLY MENU

WEDNESDAY

Breakfast	Lunch	Teatime	Dinner
Freshly squeezed grapefruit juice Fruit in season Oat flakes Skimmed milk + Brewer's yeast	Oysters Prawns Seaweed salad Wholemeal bread Water Glass of wine Espresso coffee + segment of dark chocolate (+70%) *(Optional)*	Hot chocolate with skimmed milk	Turkey leg Haricot beans with a trickle of olive oil Green salad Yoghurt, walnuts Water Glass of wine

THURSDAY

Breakfast	Lunch	Teatime	Dinner
Freshly squeezed lemon juice Fruit in season Sugar-free muesli 1 yoghurt Wheatgerm Coffee or tea	Grated raw carrots Raw red cabbage Entrecôte steak Spinach Yoghurt Water Glass of wine Espresso coffee + segment of dark chocolate (+70%) *(Optional)*	Green tea Almonds + dried apricots	Fish soup Tofu Lentil salad Cheese Wholemeal bread Water Glass of wine

PREVENTION OF CARDIOVASCULAR DISEASE WEEKLY MENU

FRIDAY

Breakfast	Lunch	Teatime	Dinner
Freshly squeezed orange juice Fruit in season Wholemeal bread Sugar-free jam Skimmed milk + Brewer's yeast Tea or coffee	Leak salad Red mullet Broccoli Cheese Wholemeal bread Water Glass of wine Espresso coffee + segment of dark chocolate (+70%) *(Optional)*	Green tea Soya milk product	Split pea soup Tomatoes stuffed with mushroom filling Soft white cheese (0% fat) + sugar- free jam

SATURDAY

Breakfast	Lunch	Teatime	Dinner
Freshly squeezed grapefruit juice Fruit in season Sugar-free muesli 1 yoghurt + wheatgerm Coffee or tea	Palmtree hearts Filet of whiting in a buttered bag Braised fennel Garlic Cheese Wholemeal bread Water Glass of wine Espresso coffee + segment of dark chocolate (+70%) *(Optional)*	Green tea Yoghurt	Cauliflower salad Black pudding Celery purée Dried figs Water Glass of wine

PREVENTION OF CARDIOVASCULAR DISEASE WEEKLY MENU

SUNDAY

Breakfast	Lunch	Teatime	Dinner
Freshly squeezed lemon juice Fruit in season 1 yoghurt Brewer's yeast Hot chocolate with skimmed milk	Foie gras + wholemeal bread toast Grille sole Aubergine purée Cheese Chocolate + vanilla bavarois Water 2 glasses of wine Espresso coffee (Optional)	Green tea Tart	Fish soup Stuffed mushrooms Yoghurt Water

5 How to live with diabetes

In France, 2.5% of the population suffer with diabetes. This percentage is far too high but considerably lower than that which we find in Anglo-Saxon countries, particularly the United States.

In fact there are two type of diabetes, quite different from each other.

Insulin-dependent diabetes (Type I)

This form of diabetes needs to be treated with injections of insulin, as the pancreas is no longer able to produce this hormone. It is, in fact, an auto-immune disease caused by the pancreas starting to produce antibodies that destroy its insulin-secreting cells.

The elderly suffering from this disease will have been aware of it for a long time, because normally it appears when we are young. As the years go by, particularly if it is not carefully regulated, many complications can arise that will adversely affect life expectancy:

• Lesions to small and large blood vessels (atheromata) that can result in blindness, angina pectoris, myocardial infarction, impotence, arteritis and blood pressure.

• Neural lesions (polyneuritits, erection problems).

• Hypoglycaemia leading to coma.

Fat diabetes, non-insulin-dependent diabetes (Type II)

This is the most frequently occurring form of the disease and affects 15 to 20% of those over sixty. It is usually discovered during a physical check-up conducted on a patient with a urinary, chest or skin infection.

Initially, Type II diabetes can be regulated by:

• losing weight if there is a weight problem, which is often the case

• following an appropriate diet

• taking appropriate medication.

This form of diabetes is characterised by hyperinsulinism and insulin-resistance - which is to say that despite insulin being secreted, blood sugar levels only decline slowly because the body cannot readily recognise the presence of insulin.

Insulin-resistance - the prime cause of diabetes - is brought about by:

• An inherited predisposition, in more than 80% of cases.

• A diet containing too many carbohydrates with a high glycaemic index. After a few years, this will trigger hyperinsulinism - leading to the onset of insulin-resistance and even give rise to a transmissible inherited characteristic, where the acquired becomes the innate.

• Hormone abnormalities.

• A sedentary lifestyle.

Dietary programme for diabetics

Type I diabetes

Because someone suffering with Type I diabetes will have sorted out their diet a long time ago, there is little further to add. Dietary recommendations are broadly the same as those given to Type II diabetics (see below), with the following exceptions:

• always eat about 15 to 20 minutes after an insulin injection

• divide food intake into four meals

• eat at regular times

• ensure you eat sufficient carbohydrates at each meal, since having a meal with no carbohydrates is the same as skipping a meal.

Type II diabetes

These are the dietary rules to follow:

- meals should be structured (three or four a day)

- never skip a meal

- select carbohydrates with a low glycaemic index, to reduce hyperglycaemia and hyperinsulinism

- choose good fats, particularly olive oil, and keep saturated fatty acids to a minimum

- eat more vegetable protein (soya, dried vegetables)

- include a selection of antioxidants

- ensure a good supply of vitamin B1 and chrome by eating Brewer's yeast

- select food rich in magnesium

- drink plenty of liquid, avoiding combinations of sugar and alcohol (beer, kir, port, muscat, gin and tonic).

A good diet is, of course, of fundamental importance, but a healthy lifestyle also has its place. So avoid smoking, stress and sitting too long in your armchair.

However, diet is not the only problem affecting a diabetic: other parameters should also be considered, such as undernourishment, loneliness, depression, lack of strength, inability to chew and loss of independence.

Foods to select for both diets

Green vegetables

Crudités, salads (watercress)

Mushrooms

Oleaginous fruit: walnuts, hazelnuts, almonds

Soya and its derivatives

Fresh fruit with its skin

Fresh fruit juice

Dark chocolate (more than 70% cocoa)

Sugar-free jam (NB – sugar or dextrose occurs naturally in grapejuice)

Pulses: haricot beans, lentils, split peas

Milk products without fat

Unrefined oats, rice, semolina

Pastas and bread made with wholemeal or unrefined flour

Brewer's yeast, wheatgerm

Sugar-free cereals

Garden peas

Fish

Shellfish

Poultry (without skin)

Rabbit

Eggs

Olive oil

Wine (2 glasses per day).

6 Alleviate rheumatic pains

Under the vague heading of rheumatism are in fact hidden several illnesses that are of particular interest to those over sixty:

- osteoporosis

- osteomalacia

- inflammatory rheumatism

- degenerative osteoarthritis

- gout.

OSTEOPOROSIS

Even though this illness is very widespread, only 36% of those interviewed were familiar with the term osteoporosis. It is characterised by an abnormal reduction in bone mass with regard to the age of the subject. It compromises the mechanical strength of the bones, even in the case of normal activities like walking. It can give rise to pain, but those suffering from it are exposed to a very real risk of bone fracture.

Bone is not an inert substance. It is constantly subject to a process of construction and destruction in order to maintain optimum strength. Should an imbalance appear between these two processes, then the bone tissue will lose mass and the bones will become brittle.

It should be remembered that bone mass is built up during childhood and stops about the age of fifteen in the case of a girl and seventeen in the case of a boy. This shows how important it is to ensure an adequate intake of calcium during childhood and adolescence, as well as during pregnancy and when women are breastfeeding. Between the ages of twenty to thirty, a simple consolidation of bone mass takes place.

From the age of forty onwards, the balance becomes slightly negative and bone mass begins to reduce due to ageing. However, the rate of deterioration will vary according to sex and bone type. Between the ages of 30 and 80, the spongy bone of a man will lose about 27% of its mass at a constant rate. On the other hand, in the case of a woman, bone loss accelerates rapidly after the menopause if there is no hormone treatment. At the age of 80, a woman will have lost about 40% of her spongy bone mass.

The two types of osteoporosis

Type I

This form occurs in the ten years that follow the onset of the menopause, if no hormone replacement therapy is undertaken.

Osteoporosis is translated into back pain, compression of the spinal column and loss of body height, which explains why women shrink and stoop after the age of sixty. But the permanent risk remains that of fracture in the case of a fall.

In France, more than 10 million women are past the menopause and each year 310,000 new "candidates" join the ranks.

Type II

This is an illness that hits both sexes, but twice as many women as men. It only starts around the age of seventy and is responsible for fractures to the neck of the thighbone.

Two factors are involved in this osteoporosis:

• a decline in the activity of the cells that ensure bone formation

• an increase in parathormone (a hormone produced by the parathyroid) caused by a lack of vitamin D (due to insufficient exposure to the sun).

Each year there are about 50,000 fractures of this type, of which 10% lead to death and 30% to mobility problems, which can give rise to nutritional imbalances.

Take your bearings

Taking a sample of blood to measure calcium levels will not indicate the presence of osteoporosis. Today we use a scanner to measure bone density.

As they approach the age of fifty, women in France can have a free examination on the National Health Service, to assess bone density and the risk of future fractures. If need be, the percentage of fatty and lean mass as well as water in the body can be calculated at the same time.

If this examination is not undertaken at the time of the menopause, it can be conducted later, when osteoporosis becomes a serious risk approaching the age of seventy.

Factors involved in osteoporosis

The genetic factor

It appears to be very strong, though this is not to say we cannot take steps to try and prevent it occurring.

Lack of calcium

Nutritional studies conducted on children and adolescents are not very reassuring, as average calcium intake is woefully inadequate.

Various studies have shown that even the elderly rarely achieve the recommended intake of 1,500mg of calcium per day. This is particularly regrettable as many of these people were children or adolescents during the Second World War, when we know there were nutritional deficiencies.

Lack of vitamin D

We mentioned earlier that vitamin D is essential for the proper absorption of calcium. It comes from food, but mainly from the synthesis that takes place in skin when exposed to the rays of the sun. A study conducted in 1922, showed that more than 70% of the elderly in retirement homes or institutions suffered from vitamin D deficiency. Not only was vitamin D lacking in their diet but also, more importantly, cutaneous synthesis was very low because even the fit were very rarely exposed to the sun.

It is precisely this lack of exposure to the sun that is principally responsible for fractures in long bones and at the neck of the femur.

Lack of hormonal contraception

The pill is oestro-progestogen and oestrogens stimulate the bone and reduce the calcium loss that theoretically would start at the age of thirty. It has been shown that women of thirty-five taking the pill have a bone density 1% higher than those who do not follow this form of contraception. And of course, our grandmothers knew nothing about the pill.

Top women athletes do not have their periods and normally do not take oral contraceptives. Despite their intense physical activity, the osteoporotic process starts very early and their bones become disturbingly brittle. After the age of sixty, these women become a risk group.

Untreated menopause

Today it is well shown that hormone treatment for the menopause, desirable in limiting the signs of ageing and preventing cardiovascular disease, enables us to slow down the evolution of osteoporosis quite considerably. This is why we must be as vigilant as possible in cases of early menopause, whether caused spontaneously or by surgical intervention, as in the case of an hysterectomy.

Lack of physical activity

Regular physical activity is a protection against osteoporosis. A study conducted on cross-country runners with an average age of fifty showed an increase of 20% in the mass of long bones and 10% in those of the spine when compared to a group of inactive people of the same age. Bone appeared to be more sensitive to the frequency rather than the intensity of the exercise to which it was subjected.

Lack of physical activity, staying indoors or immobility, caused by physical handicap or having broken a bone, will considerably increase the osteoporotic process in those over sixty years of age.

Being thin

Thin women are more exposed to osteoporosis at the time of their menopause.

The androgens produced by the adrenal glands of plump women can be partially transformed into oestrogens, affording them a certain measure of protection.

Tobacco addiction

On average, the menopause arrives eight months earlier in the case of occasional female smokers, and a year and a half in the case of daily smokers.

In addition, an important and largely unknown fact is that after the menopause, tobacco addiction undermines the positive effects of replacement hormones on bones and contributes to development osteoporosis. Moreover, by causing blood vessels to constrict and reducing cell exchanges, tobacco addiction accelerates ageing in general and the skin in particular.

Taking medicine

Cortisone taken over an extended period, say for asthma or inflammatory rheumatism, will encourage the onset of osteoporosis.

Dietary imbalances

In addition to a low-calorie diet, lack of calcium and vitamin D, too much alcohol or coffee (more than 5 cups a day) - all contribute to the onset of osteoporosis.

The dietetic of osteoporosis

After hormonal and nutritional preventative measures have been taken, osteoporosis must be treated when detected.

Classical therapies incorporate the following elements:

- calcium
- vitamin D3
- phosphorus
- fluorine
- calcitonin
- diphosphonate.

Ensure correct calcium intake

For elderly people, calcium intake should be 1,500mg per day - particularly for women, who are more vulnerable to osteoporosis than men.

FOODS RICH IN CALCIUM

in mg per 100g or 100ml

Brewer's yeast	2,000
Gruyere	1,200
Other cheeses	800 to 1000
Prunes	800
Sardines (with bones)	400
Condensed milk	300
Eggs	300
Milk chocolate	220
Parsley, cress	200
Dried fruit	200
Natural yoghurt	170
Soft white cheese	125
Milk	110
Cauliflower, broccoli	100
Black chocolate	100
Mussels, oysters	100
Prawns	100
Bread (unrefined flour)	50

Water from the tap can be a good source of calcium if it is "hard". (Tap water in Paris, for example, contains 100mg/l.) The concentration of calcium per litre of mineral water is as follows:

- 600mg for Vittel Hépar
- 78mg for Evian.

This translates roughly into 1,000mg (or 1g) of calcium in:

- 1 litre of milk
- 1.5 litres of Vittel Hépar
- 10 glasses of Parisian water
- 12 litres of Evian
- 80g of Comté cheese
- 100g of Gruyere cheese
- 150g of Dutch cheese
- 650g of soft white cheese.

To improve the absorption of calcium, intake should be divided up over the course of the day.

People with major cardiovascular problems, should perhaps avoid having milk as its proteins may favour the formation of atheromata on the internal walls of the larger arteries. On the other hand, as there is no correlation between eating cheese and the incidence of cardiovascular disease, it seems likely the modification undergone by cheese protein during fermentation suppresses any atherogenic risk.

We also know that an intolerance to lactose (milk carbohydrate) is generally caused by a deficiency in the digestive enzyme lactase and that it can give rise to the formation of cataracts. It is preferable to eat products that do not contain lactose, which is the case after milk has been fermented. This is why we should avoid milk, soft white cheeses or petit-suisse cheeses, but must eat fermented milk products like yoghurt and cheese.

Instead of eating 50g of Comté cheese at lunch, try eating a yoghurt at breakfast, as a snack between meals and at dinner; this will already give you a daily calcium intake slightly in excess of 1,200mg.

Ensure a good intake of phosphorus

Like calcium, phosphorus can be found mainly in milk products. A daily intake of 1,500mg is recommended, as ideally the intake ratio of calcium to phosphorus should equal unity.

FOODS RICH IN PHOSPHORUS

in mg per 100g or 100ml

Brewer's yeast	3,000
Cheese	200 to 800
Soya seed	600
Chocolate	280
Fish, meat	150 to 250
Condensed milk	200
Eggs	200
Bread (unrefined flour)	180
Yoghurt	120
White rice	100
White bread (refined flour)	100
Broccoli	80

Ensure an adequate concentration of vitamin D

When exposed to the activity of the sun, our skin synthesises vitamin D. Exposing our hands for fifteen minutes at least three days a week between 11 am and 2pm will be sufficient to meet our requirements. A complementary intake of nutrients is always useful.

FOODS CONTAINING VITAMIN D

Cod liver oil	Tuna
Sardines	Mushrooms
Pork	Chicken
Animal liver	Butter
Cheese	Wheatgerm

Certain nutrients prevent osteoporosis

- Vitamin C: scurvy, which occurs in the case of extreme deficiency, accompanies osteoporosis.

- Vitamin B6: a lack of this vitamin encourages osteoporosis. We now know that 85% of those over sixty have an intake of vitamin B6 which is below the Recommended Daily Allowance (RDA).

Certain nutrients taken in excess encourage osteoporosis

- Vitamin A: avoid taking supplements blindly. Choose complementary foods whenever possible.

- Proteins: the RDA is 1g per kilo of body weight per day - but no more, otherwise you will need more calcium to replace what has been lost through increased urination.

- Coffee: do not exceed more than five cups a day, particularly those women with a calcium intake lower than 600mg per day. Moreover, milk added to coffee will inhibit calcium absorption.

- Foods rich in oxalates: which will trap calcium in an insoluble oxalate (spinach, sorrel, beetroot, rhubarb, red and white currants, and gooseberry).

- Distilled alcohol (spirits).

OSTEOPOROSIS

Foods to choose	Foods to avoid in quantity
Brewer's yeast	Spinach
Cheeses (particularly Comté and Gruyere)	Sorrel
Wheatgerm	Beetroot
Tuna and sardines	Red and white currants
Shellfish	Gooseberries
Chicken	Coffee + milk
Eggs	
Animal liver	
Watercress, cauliflower, broccoli	
Parsley	
Mushrooms	
Prunes	
Dried fruit: apricots, figs	
Mineral waters (Vittel Hépar)	
Chocolate (+ 70% cocoa)	

OSTEOMALACIA

This is an illness that is often ignored but which deserves careful study, as it can dramatically affect the lives of those afflicted. Treatment, however, is quite simple.

It is the adult form of rickets, involving the demineralisation of the skeleton, which results in fissures appearing in the bones.

Causes

Osteomalacia is due to a vitamin D deficiency that causes a reduction in the calcium/phosphorus ratio.

This lack of vitamin D can have several causes:

• inadequate exposure to the sun

• dietary deficiency (no milk products, fats or eggs)

• poor absorption of vitamin D (excessive use of digestive palliatives)

• chronic renal malfunction.

Symptoms

There are many signs associated with osteomalacia:

• Pelvic pains, particularly in the groin, spreading to the front of the thighs. These pains are accompanied by a lack of movement in the hips: the gait becomes slow and hesitant and the steps short. The sufferer looks for means of support and sometimes believes the condition is due to a lack of muscular strength.

These problems with walking, perhaps to be expected among the elderly, should immediately make us think in terms of osteomalacia.

• Occasional thoracic pains, awakened by pressure on the ribs.

• Physical and psychological asthenia, sometimes accompanied by loss of weight. In the absence of any treatment, the sufferer runs the risk of moving less and less, and of not being able to get up anymore. With treatment, within a few days the mobility problems disappear and the patient starts walking normally.

How do we diagnose the illness?

Taking a blood sample is not a great help, even though we may be able to find low phosphorous levels in the blood. On the other hand, X-ray photographs will show characteristic fissures particularly in the pelvic region. At a more advanced stage, we might even have a straightforward fracture. Moreover, the signs of osteoporosis that normally coexist with osteomalacia are also visible.

However, every attempt should be made to diagnose the condition as soon as possible, because by the time we detect fissures the condition is already well advanced.

Treatment

Vitamin D is administered in drops or by injection. The pains disappear in less than a month and, if fissures exist, they will be filled within two or three months. After this, it is important to ensure an adequate supply of vitamin D in order to avoid a recurrence.

INFLAMMATORY RHEUMATISMS

Except in the case of gout, researchers are unfortunately not very interested in the interactions between diet and rheumatic diseases. However, rheumatoid polyarthritis has benefited from a few attempts at nutritional therapy. This illness starts about the age of forty, but it can be seen to develop in people over the age of sixty.

Rheumatoid polyarthritis is an inflammatory rheumatism that affects 1.5% of the French. It develops by painful rheumatic attacks that cause stiffening of the joints with important after-effects over the years.

Dietary experiments have been undertaken recently to calm the inflammatory attacks and even to achieve longer periods of remission.

Fasting

In the event of a very painful attack, the patient may be subjected to seven days of fasting under very strict medical supervision. The patient is allowed to eat only vegetable soup.

Personalised exclusion diet

Twenty foods are withdrawn from the diet and then re-introduced one by one every two days, taking a note of possible reactions, such as pain, swelling and joint stiffness. Foods that appear to be responsible for any attacks of the illness, are permanently eliminated.

The test foods are as follows:

• sweetcorn, wheat, oats, rye

• soya

- peanuts

- pork

- beef

- lamb

- orange, lemon, grapefruit

- tomato

- sugar

- butter

- eggs

- cheese, milk

- coffee.

Statistics show that:

- 37% of patients are affected by 1 to 5 foods

- 37% of patients are affect by 6 to 10 foods

- 26% of patients are affected by more than 10 foods.

The Seignalet diet

- All cereals are excluded from the diet, with the exception of rice.

- Milk and all its derivatives are also excluded.

- Raw products are introduced, including fish and meat.

- Oils derived from cold, first pressings are introduced, with particular importance being given to oil of evening primrose.

A year-long trial of this diet involving 130 people gave a positive result in 80% of the cases.

Intake of protein

A diet that is too rich in protein, encourages inflammatory outbreaks of the disease.

Fish oils

These will have an anti-inflammatory effect, but only if they are taken in sufficient amounts - about twenty capsules daily.

However, these doses have the drawback of modifying blood coagulation factors, exposing the elderly to the risk of a cerebral haemorrhage.

In conclusion, we could say that these investigations represent an interesting line of research, but the results are still too fragmentary to draw any definite conclusions. Be that as it may, the recommendations are difficult to apply in view of the constraints imposed by the limited choice of authorised foods.

OSTEOARTHRITIS

This is certainly one of the least well known of rheumatic diseases, as well as one of the most frequent. Moreover, it draws in its wake a formidable selection of generally accepted ideas.

It involves the damage to the cartilage of a joint deformed at its bony extremities. It is an ailment that is rare before the age of fifty, but very common after the age of sixty. It particularly affects the hands, knees, hips and the spinal column. It is too often thought to be the result of the ageing process, when it is well and truly a fully fledged disease.

The causes

At the moment these are unclear, even if certain mechanical constraints often seem to play a determining role.

In fact it is clear that being overweight adds to the pressure being placed on the joints. Common sense therefore demands that those beginning to suffer from the disease should lose weight, to reduce the weight bearing on the joints and the resulting mechanical pain.

Remedies

The beneficial effect of antioxidants (vitamins C and E, betacarotene, selenium, zinc, copper and polyphenols) has often been referred to, without ever having been proven.

As silicon and manganese feature in the composition of cartilage, an adequate intake of these elements would seem to offer a reasonable solution.

FOODS RICH IN SILICON

Green vegetables

Tomatoes with skin

Wholemeal bread or bread made from unrefined flour

Brown rice

Radishes

Horsetail tisane

FOODS RICH IN MANGANESE

Walnuts

Tea

Ginger

Cloves

Cereals

Wheatgerm

Spinach and other green vegetables

Almonds

Fresh fruit

Copper, selenium and fish oils may help to combat inflammatory attacks.

GOUT (HYPERURECAEMIA)

Gout is the principal complication arising from a high level of uric acid in the blood (hyperuricaemia). During a sharp attack, it manifests itself in a joint (big toe, knee, wrist), triggering an inflammatory attack.

Each day, a normal, healthy person will produce 600mg of uric acid, which is either synthesised by the body or results from the nucleic degradation occurring in cells that are being renewed: 200mg of this uric acid is eliminated in faeces and 400mg in urine.

The average level of uric acid in the blood of a man is 55mg/l and this figure does not change very much with age. We talk of hyperuricaemia when this figure goes beyond the critical threshold of 70mg/l. About 17% of all Frenchmen suffer with this condition.

The average level of uric acid in the blood of women is 40mg/l and 45mg/l after the menopause. This level becomes critical when it exceeds 60mg per litre, though only 3% of French women are affected.

Causes

There is either an excess production of uric acid, through dietary excesses for example, or there is a reduced elimination of uric acid due to renal insufficiency. In 95% of cases, there is an hereditary cause. However, excess uric acid can be triggered by:

• *illness*

  obesity

  blood disease (leukaemia)

  Bierner's anaemia (lack of vitamin B12)

  malfunction of the parathyroid glands

  diabetes with ketoaciduria

  cardiac insufficiency

  renal insufficiency

  thyroid insufficiency

  lactic acidosis

- *medication*

  diuretics

  aspirin

  anti-tubercular treatment

  chemotherapy for cancers

- *overexertion*

  particularly in cases of extended physical exertion, involving the destruction of muscle cells and red blood cells (e.g. running the marathon)

- *diet restrictions*

  fasting

  very low-calorie diets.

Complications

- Gout is the most frequent manifestation.
- Uric lithiasis which can give rise to urinary infections and nephritic colic (kidney stones), particularly when urine levels are low due to not drinking enough or sweating heavily.
- Renal insufficiency can eventually result in a total deterioration of the kidneys, requiring kidney replacement.
- Cardiovascular complications (arrhythmia, coronary risk, angina, myocardial infarction, high blood pressure).

Treatment

As well as appropriate medical treatment, the excess of uric acid can be regulated by dietary means.

- Reduce any excess weight, as it increases any risk by 20 to 30%.

- Undergo natural diuretic treatment, perhaps at a spa. This will entail increasing the volume of urine by drinking a lot of water with a low acid content.

- Drink mineral water containing a small amount of bicarbonate and freshly squeezed lemon juice. Milk products also contain acid neutralising alkalies.

- Reduce alcohol intake: eliminate the consumption of spirits, white wine, port and Burgundy wine, and with regard to the rest, they should be drunk in moderation (no more than two glasses per day).

- Reduce protein intake to 1g per kilo of body weight. This applies particularly to "sporty" types who want to "build up their muscles".

- Avoid eating foods containing high levels of uric acid and purines, such as:

  Sweetbreads

  Anchovies

  Sardines

  Brain

  Liver, kidneys

  Herring

  Fish eggs

  Pig's trotters

  Tongue

  Sausage

  Tripe

  Veal head

  Gelatine

  Meat broth.

- Eat with moderation the following foods which contain uric acid and purines:

  Trout, carp

  Game

Turkey

Piglet

Air-dried meats

Shellfish

Lentils

Spinach, sorrel

Asparagus

Choucroute (sauerkraut), fermented cauliflower

Mushrooms

Cheeses

Chocolate, coffee, tea.

7 Suppress constipation and colitis

We all have our little weaknesses and ways of reacting at the psychosomatic level. There are many people who focus their anguish on their colon and so become so-called "faecal obsessives". Every day, the frequency, importance, consistency and general aspect of their motions become their favourite subject of conversation.

CONSTIPATION

If we want to be as non-prosaic and as technical as possible, we must define constipation as delayed evacuation associated with faecal dehydration. Some have defined constipation as three or fewer stools a week.

The norm is between three and seven stools a week. It is probably good to have one stool a day, but it is not at all obligatory. Too many people worry if their daily rhythm is not strictly adhered to.

Different types of constipation

Recent, unexpected constipation

This should cause us to consider the possibility of colonic or rectal cancer, particularly if the motions contain blood. Your doctor should assess the situation himself or have it assessed by others, so that he can make the appropriate diagnosis.

It is truly a disease caused by civilisation, by our modern diet where we eat too much saturated fat and not enough fibre. In equatorial Africa, in the bush where the diet is very rich in cereals and poor in meat, these cancers are unknown. In France, on the other hand, they are responsible for 15,000 deaths a year - a fact that should remind us that a suspect constipation should never be ignored.

Persistent or chronic constipation

In this case, we are dealing with someone who has always had a sluggish intestinal action and this long-standing problem has been accentuated by:

- lack of physical activity, perhaps a mobility problem

- medication: neuroleptics, antidepressants, atropines

- bladder deficiency

- sugar addiction

- lack of alimentary bulk or bolus

- insufficient liquid intake.

This form of constipation can be caused by a lack of muscular tone (atonic), resulting in an inflated belly, or spasmodic and accompanied by acute pain - as with colitis. In both cases, a sensible diet and a healthy lifestyle will rectify the situation.

Rectal dyschezia

This barbarous term is applied to a condition where the patient has no reflex bowel movement. In addition to general dietary advice, this form of constipation may require a complete re-education of the evacuant reflex - for example, by applying biofeedback techniques taught by a specially trained kinetotherapist.

Eat properly and avoid constipation

- Try to be regular, choosing a time when you are likely to feel bowel activity – for example, after a meal.

- Drink at least 1.5 litres of liquid per day. Water is perfect, but you can also take fresh fruit juice (with pulp) or prune juice. Chicory is slightly laxative and may be considered, particularly as we should avoid drinking too much astringent coffee and tea. On the other hand, contrary to received wisdom, we find that chocolate does not, in fact, cause constipation.

• Increase faecal bulk by having a diet rich in fibre:

  – fresh fruit (with skin)

  – freshly squeezed fruit juice, with the pulp (lemon, orange, grapefruit)

  – stewed fruit compote

  – fruit jam, preferably without sugar but containing soluble fibre in the form of pectin

  – raw vegetables and salads, dressed with olive oil

  – cooked vegetables (mashed, if required)

  – vegetable soup

  – cereals, preferably unrefined

  – cereals with bran

  – unrefined foods (bread, rice, pasta, semolina)

  – dried vegetables (lentils, beans, split peas, haricot and kidney beans), mashed if necessary

  – Brewer's yeast (1 coffee-spoon daily, in yoghurt) rich in vitamin B1, which has a tonic effect on the intestinal wall

  – as a last resort, 1 tablespoon of bran (from organically cultivated cereals).

  However, for those that are not used to a fibre-rich diet, the change should be implemented **very** gradually, to allow the colon time to adapt and to avoid provoking an attack of colitis.

• Stimulate the action of the gall bladder.

  Bile actively accelerates the passage of food through the intestines, and its secretion can be increased by taking the following on an empty stomach:

  – a tablespoon of olive oil, followed by the juice of one lemon

  – a sachet of sorbitol

  – or some meat broth at mealtime.

  Oil of paraffin should be not be taken – it is derived from hydrocarbons that interfere with the intestinal absorption of micronutrients and contain no vitamins or essential fatty acids.

• Regulate colic flora by eating a couple of yoghurts each day.

- Develop a healthier lifestyle:

  - take a daily walk lasting at least one hour (unless you have mobility problems). Swim or cycle if possible.

  - do exercises to strengthen the abdominal muscles that need to contract to ensure intestinal evacuation

  - stop taking laxatives - these can give rise to "laxative illness", a very severe condition combining colitis, dehydration and potassium starvation, to produce cramps and possibly arrhythmia. It also seems to be responsible for the onset of intestinal cancers.

  - use a gentle mucilage or glycerine suppositories for a brief period

  - eliminate all medication likely to cause constipation. This can pose problems, however, if the patient is being treated for a psychiatric disorder.

Treating constipation is all the more important as indirectly it helps to prevent:

- gastro-oesophageal reflux

- hiatus hernias and their associated illnesses

- haemorrhoids

- varicose veins in the legs

A fibre-rich diet prevents or alleviates diverticular colitis, which affects one in three of the elderly. It is an illness of the sigmoid colon, where little bulges or sacks (diverticules) form on the wall of the colon. They are susceptible to inflammation or infection, and sometimes form the bed for a digestive cancer, though - like polyps, which are also common - they can regress with a diet rich in fibre.

COLITIS

This is also known as "spasmodic colopathy" or "irritable bowl syndrome". It is in reality a hypersensitivity of the large intestine to fermentation and alimentary fibre. It then becomes the object of painful spasms or of irritation along its wall.

During the phases of intense irritation, a fibre-free diet becomes a temporary necessity. The recommended diet is then:

- normal, white rice (not sticky)

- fish, steamed or poached in a court-bouillon

- boiled eggs

- white pasta

- sieved vegetable soup

- steamed chicken

- vegetables: cooked and liquidized

- vegetable mousse (broccoli or spinach, for example)

- peeled, cooked fruit

- still mineral water

- olive oil

- lemons

- chicory.

The following foods should be avoided:

- milk products (milk, butter, cheese, yoghurt)

- fatty meats

- fried foods

- unrefined cereals

- pulses (lentils, dried beans, peas).

Those suffering with colitis will tend to exclude all fibre from their diet. This is a mistake. After the attacks, fibre should be reintroduced into the diet, very progressively. After a week of excluding fibre from the diet, cooked green vegetables (leeks, French beans, broccoli) should be reintroduced together with cooked fruit (apples). Then, still very progressively, raw food (vegetables, salads, fruit) should be reintroduced into the diet. In the end, we can start eating unrefined foods (pastas, rice, cereals, bread and sweetcorn) in small quantities, increasing the portions day by day. The diet will also have to include pulses.

Charcoal or clay may be taken to alleviate pain or absorb gas. In the case of diverticulitis, fibre must be included in the diet to avoid infections and prevent the condition becoming cancerous.

8 Stimulate your defences

THE IMMUNE SYSTEM

The role of the immune system is to protect the body from disease caused by the invasion of micro-organisms (bacteria, viruses, fungi and parasites). This role is guaranteed by white blood corpuscles (leukocytes) and a certain number of other cells.

These cells are scattered throughout the body, but are located mainly in the lymphoid organs (bone marrow, spleen and lymphatic ganglions). They occur in large numbers at potential entry sites for pathogenic micro-organisms - in the mucous membranes of the intestine and the lungs. Their role is therefore to organise an immune response in order to eliminate pathogens or minimise the damage they can cause.

Following entry into the body of a foreign substance recognised as being undesirable, called an antigen, the immune system triggers two types of response:

1 a "humoral" response, producing antibodies from lymphocytes originating from B cells

2 a "cellular" response by lymphocytes originating from T cells, whose role is to capture the antigens.

In a way, it is like mobilising a real army against enemy aggression - whence the phrase "immunological defences" to describe this "rapid reaction force". Such a concept makes it easier to understand that when these means of defence are powerful, the intruder will be easily repelled and good health ensured. However, when these immune defences are weak, the body will be vulnerable to illness and health will be poor.

There are people who catch a cold several times a year, regardless of the season and in the mildest of draughts. There are others - perhaps even seventy years old - who take a dip in the North Sea in January with no problem at all. The difference between the two lies in their immunological defences.

We are surrounded by microbes and, contrary to what is often thought, they have an important role to play in our existence, for they form part of nature's biological balance. To disinfect everything in sight is a mistake. Not only does it weaken our immune defences by depriving them of their permanent role (which keeps them in peak form to deal with a heavy attack), but also indirectly it allows resistant colonies of micro-organisms to develop that even a healthy body will have difficulty in combating.

Upsetting or weakening our immune system will result in:

- Infections: over the age of sixty, these will be mainly urinary or pulmonary (bronchitis, pneumonia), flu, secondary infection of wounds (leg ulcers, bedsores, wounds on the feet of diabetics, post-operative complications).

- Poor protection (against flu for example), despite vaccinations.

- Slow healing of bone fractures or muscular recovery (after being confined to bed).

- Auto-immune illnesses. In these extreme cases, the immune system secretes antibodies against the cells of its own body. This happens particularly with cancer, diabetes type I, rheumatoid polyarthritis, multiple sclerosis.

These illnesses are not particularly associated with age but they are often found in advanced forms among the elderly.

We will discover in this chapter that, without being exactly a panacea, diet is a determining factor in keeping immune defences at an optimum level. It is, in any case, the only factor that we can use effectively when dealing with an inherited weakness in combating the illness.

Stimulating the immune system

When a body is subjected to attack - invaded, let us say, by a germ - there are several possible scenarios:

1 If the means of defence are operational, the body will bring its immune system into operation. The lymphocytes will do their work and the infection will not be apparent or, at very least, it will be quickly checked. At most, we

will have a sore throat that will last a few hours and some glands in the neck that will swell up a little (these glands are made of lymphatic tissue rich in lymphocytes).

2 This is a sign that the body has an effective immune system, enabling it to drive out the enemy or, at the very least, stop it in its tracks.

3 The body's means of defence have lost their strength and need to be stimulated. It is at this point that biostimulation techniques like homeopathy and acupuncture can play a part.

4 We talk of "biostimulation" because we act on functions existing in the body that are momentarily faltering. This form of stimulation encourages internal secretion of chemical transmitters in larger quantities (endorphins, cortisol, catecholamines, etc.) and is a lash of the whip enabling the defences to do their work. Giving biostimulation before or after this stage will have no effect.

5 The body is no longer able to play its part because its immune defences are too feeble. It is unable to control the action of the germ and cannot check the infection. We must therefore act on its behalf. This is the role of allopathy - more precisely, antibiotics and anti-inflammatory drugs that do not act with the body but rather in its place.

6 At this stage, any stimulation of the immune system would be in vain. Just as it is absurd to whip an exhausted horse to make it go faster, so is it pointless to stimulate a body "at the end of its tether".

7 The affected organ is not only ineffective, but can become dangerous by infecting the rest of the body. It is at this point that surgery is used to remove the damaged tissue.

When he comes face to face with a patient, the skill of the doctor is to determine the background to the case. Certainly small infections have no pressing need for antibiotics, which often do more harm than good. For just as we do not use an atomic bomb to kill a fly, for it would clearly cause collateral damage, so we do not employ antibiotics that would inevitably prevent the immune defence system from being ready to play its role confronting a more dangerous enemy in the future.

On the other hand, if we were confronted with scenario 3 or perhaps 4, it would be rash to intervene only with mild medicines for reasons that are more philosophical than medical.

In this scheme of things, how will the dietary factor work? In scenario 1, the dietary method would play a preventative role in maintaining the body "in full possession of its faculties". In scenario 2, the dietary approach could contribute by bringing the system back onto an even keel, rapidly correcting any deficiencies undermining the immune system. In the other cases, it could accompany therapy, making a better recovery possible.

EAT PROPERLY TO AVOID INFECTIONS

Diet plays a cardinal role in controlling immune response. In fact, some dietary deficiencies help perpetuate weaknesses in the immune system, just as some foods can reinforce defences. But we shall also see that the treatment of food, both domestic and industrial, is important too.

Eat protein

An inadequate protein intake is one of the main factors contributing to a poor immune defence. Immune activity is correlated to the level of albumen in the blood. Any lack of protein in the diet will expose us to bacterial, viral or mycotic infection.

We should therefore eat the following regularly:

- eggs, mainly boiled (on average, one every other day), making sure they come from free range, not industrial chickens

- fish, either raw (smoked or marinated salmon) or steamed

- meat, rare or raw (steak tartar)

- fermented cheese made from unpasteurised milk and all cheeses with washed rinds

- soya milk (calcium enriched).

Give up milk and fresh milk products (soft, white cheese and petit-suisse cheeses), with the exception of yoghurt.

Calorie content

An additional 500 kcal per day is often sufficient to restore proper immunity to infection. From this we can see the inherent dangers associated with following a low-calorie diet.

Boost vitamin intake

A large number of vitamins play a part in helping the immune system to function properly - specifically vitamins A, B1, B6, B9, B2, C, D, E, and betacarotene.

To help the immune system recover, we can include the following in our diet:

- dried Brewer's yeast (6 tablets or 2 coffee spoons per day)

- raw carrots (organic)

- cod liver oil (3 to 4 capsules per day)

- wheatgerm oil (2 coffee spoons per day)

- chicken liver

- parsley, broccoli, lemons, oranges.

Fill up on trace elements

It has been shown that a significant lack of zinc, copper, iron and selenium leads to low resistance to infection. However, we must be careful in the way we supplement our diet: an immune deficiency occurs when we have either an excess or deficiency in zinc.

Foods to give preference to:

- oysters

- mussels, cockles and black pudding

- unrefined cereals

- fish, meat.

Choose good fats

The quality of fatty acids plays an important part in ensuring we have an effective immune response. For example, too much oxidised polysaturated fatty acid reduces immune response by depressing T lymphocytes.

This is what happens when we use delicate and unstable oils coming from a first cold pressing that have been stored in poor conditions where, perhaps, it is warm and light. They oxidise, giving a rancid taste, owing mainly to a lack in vitamin E. This is particularly the case with corn oil and sunflower oil; olive oil, on the other hand, does not suffer from these problems because it is very stable.

Eat foods that stimulate the immune system

This has been shown to happen with cabbage, cauliflower, Brussels sprouts and broccoli, whether they are eaten raw or steam-cooked - though it may be due quite simply to the high level of antioxidants they contain.

Yoghurt also seems to have quite exceptional properties: according to various studies that have been made, 200g of yoghurt per day appear to be sufficient to improve the immunity of those over fifty, and 450g per day can even stimulate the production of interferon, helping to improve the immune response of those suffering with Aids.

Attention to cooking

Different studies and experiments have confirmed that various ways of cooking can adversely affect the quality of foods and the extent to which they help maintain our immune defences.

In addition to eliminating vitamins, cooking at high temperatures (above 100°C) results in the destructuring of single molecules and the appearance of residual substances that seriously undermine the immune system. So we should eliminate foods cooked at high temperature in an oven, frying pan, pressure cooker or fryer.

For the same reasons, we are advised to eat raw foods as often as possible (vegetables and fruit in particular) or foods cooked at temperatures below 100°C - that is, in a steamer.

A healthy lifestyle

To avoid getting germs, viruses or parasites that can cause severe infections like salmonella or parasitosis, we should avoid eating foods of inferior quality that have been too long in the refrigerator or industrial foods (eggs from battery

FOODS AND PRACTICES TO HELP IMPROVE IMMUNE RESPONSE

Foods to select

Raw carrots
Cabbage, cauliflower
Broccoli, Brussels sprouts
Onion
Garlic
Boiled egg
Yoghurt
Cheeses: Roquefort, Reblochon, Tomme de Savoie
Steamed fish
Raw fish
Underdone meat, steak Tartare, Carpaccio
Fresh fruit
Radish, horseradish
Parsley, chervil
Dried Brewer's yeast
Walnuts, hazelnuts, almonds
Olive oil
Wheatgerm oil
Walnut oil
Oysters
Shellfish
Cockles
Black pudding
Rice (steam-cooked)
Wine: 2 to 3 glasses per day
Honey
Raw ham

Foods to avoid

Milk
Soft white cheese
Cheese gratin
Grills
Deep-fried foods
Braised and grilled meats
Simmered dishes
Chips and baked potatoes
White bread
White pastas
Refined sugar
Cooked ham

Recommended
Eat raw foods, steamed foods or foods cooked at low temperatures

Not recommended
Smoking
Cooking In the oven, on the barbecue or in a deep fryer

chickens, for example). Contrary to that which we said earlier, if we have any doubt about the quality of our food or we have no choice, it is better to eat these foods cooked, even if we know from elsewhere that eating raw food helps to stimulate an immune response. It is for this reason that we should be careful about eating mayonnaise and confectioner's custard if we cannot be certain they are fresh.

Guarding against too much air pollution should also be part of the programme, particularly smoking, as it has been shown that tobacco significantly reduces our ability to fight infection.

9 Nutritional safeguards against cancer

A few decades ago, everybody saw cancer as a prime cause of death. The very many studies conducted since then have tended to show that 80% of cancers are due to environmental factors and 60% of cancers in women are due to nutritional mistakes. As a general rule however, we could say that, for the French, one in every two cancers could be avoided if all the French drank in moderation and stopped smoking.

WHAT IS A CANCER?

The appearance of a cancer results from the action of different parameters linked to the environment, on a body with an inherited predisposition to the illness.

Environmental factors on the one hand, bad dietary habits on the other and the carcinogenic substances they produce constitute initiators that will result in real modifications to body cells, such that potentially they will be able to modify and proliferate themselves.

Among environmental initiators we can name:

• Nitrosamines of nitrates

• Benzopyrenes from grilled barbecue foods

• Pesticides, insecticides, herbicides, fungicides

• Aflatoxine from badly preserved peanuts

• Biphenylpolychlorates (BPC)

• Polyvinylchlorides (PVC)

• Certain heavy metals, asbestos.

But for the cells modified in this way by these initiators to start to multiply, become cancerous and form a tumour, there must be a factor that triggers the event. This event is called a promoter. Among these promoters, we find bad practices such as eating excessive amounts of meat fat, drinking too much alcohol, nicotine and high cooking temperatures.

A body cell only becomes cancerous after a chain of several abnormal sequences. The dietary factor is therefore only one link in the chain, even though it may be a main link in some cancers. As far as the immune defences of the body are concerned, the dietary factor is very important as it plays a part in regulating the development and growth of abnormal cells.

Incidence of different cancers

For people over sixty, the most frequent cancers are:

Men	Women
1. Prostate	1. Colon-rectum
2. Lungs	2. Breast
3. Colon-rectum	3. Stomach
4. Stomach	4. Uterus
5. Bladder	5. Ovaries
6. Oesophagus	
7. Pancreas	
8. Larynx	

However, in years to come, lung cancer among women is set to increase, reaching second or third position. This is due to the marked increase in tobacco addiction among women over the last thirty years.

Causes of cancer

Studies and statistics make a convincing case for indicting tobacco addiction, alcoholism, bad eating habits, pollution, certain chemical products and professional factors.

However, we should approach these matters with a certain amount of caution, because the correlation between an aggressive factor and the appearance of a cancer is always difficult to establish. Yet, having said this, the evidence accumulated over the years clearly allows us to determine which nutrients and foods are likely to encourage the appearance of a cancer as opposed to those that have a protective role.

Factors likely to encourage the appearance of a cancer

Excess weight

People who remain close to their ideal weight are less susceptible to develop cancer than the obese and particularly those who are thin. Cancers of the uterus, breast, gall bladder, prostate and colon-rectum are statistically more likely to occur to people who are 20% overweight.

Android obesity (obesity in the upper body) is more closely associated with cancer than gynecoid obesity (obesity in the lower body).

A man who is obese and eats a lot of fat runs four times the risk of contracting prostate cancer as does a man of average corpulence who eats little fat. On the other hand, undernourishment, which can make you thin but also undermines your immune defences, may well lead to the onset of cancer.

Bad fats

Too much fat in our diet (more than 40%) makes the cancers of the ovary, uterus, pancreas, prostate and especially colon and rectum, much more likely.

In fact, fats are indirectly responsible for an increased risk of cancer, because they require a much higher level of biliary acid in order to digest them through the intestines. However, perhaps the problem is less the quantity of fat but rather its nature. In fact, there are many people who think the saturated fatty acids in meat, delicatessen meats and milk products, are much more harmful than fish fats and the oils from olives and evening primrose, which they believe have a protective effect. Meat is very much in the hot seat with regards to the causes of prostate, colonic and rectal cancers.

Vegetable polyunsaturated fats coming from a first cold pressing can lead to the formation of cancer, inducing free radicals when there is a lack of antioxidants like vitamin E, owing to exposure to light and normal room temperatures. Paraffin oil should be avoided, partly because it is derived from hydrocarbons and partly because it inhibits the absorption of micronutrients in the colon, particularly antioxidants.

Some proteins

Vegetarians suffer less with cancer than omnivores, but they also tend to have a healthier lifestyle, consuming little or no alcohol or tobacco.

Recent studies seem to show that proteins from the milk of goats and cows interfere with the immune system and may contribute to the development of anti-immune diseases and cancers. However, only milk - even when skimmed - and fresh milk products, like soft white cheese and petit-suisses, seem to be involved: yoghurts and cheeses made from fermented milk straight from the cow are not involved.

Bad carbohydrates

Several studies have incriminated sugar as a contributory factor in breast, colonic and rectal cancer. If the refining process is to blame in the case of sugar, it is probable that excessive use of hyper-refined white flour will also be under suspicion one day, as it is also a carbohydrate with its fibre removed.

Too much alcohol

Regular consumption of high levels of alcohol increases the risk of contracting cancers of the mouth, tongue, pharynx, oesophagus, liver, rectum, bladder and breast.

In the liver, alcohol increases the level of cytochrome P 450, known to make various substances in the body carcinogenic. As alcohol is not itself carcinogenic but probably merely a co-carcinogen, it acts in concert with other substances, which it helps to penetrate the alimentary tract and damage the cells of the small intestine.

Some alcoholic drinks also contain carcinogenic substances, like nitrosamines in certain beers, but only drinks with an aniseed base are linked to cancers of the bladder.

On the other hand, alcohol abuse gives rise to immune deficiencies that encourage the development of cancers. We should not forget that an alcoholic has an unbalanced diet - poor in vitamins, selenium and antioxidants - which is very likely to encourage the development of cancer. However, the most formidable interaction likely to cause cancer is that between alcohol and tobacco (cancers of the ventilatory and digestive systems in the upper body).

Salted and smoked foods

Asiatic countries (China and particularly Japan) have long paid a heavy price, in the form of stomach cancer, for their practice of preserving fish by salting and smoking.

Nitrates in water

The nitrates present in water or in delicatessen meats, or any other industrial salting methods for that matter, can be transformed into carcinogenic nitrosamines in the stomach.

Chlorinated water

Studies are beginning to point the finger at chlorine by-products dissolved in drinking water for causing cancer of the kidneys and bladder. However, the specialists are not counting on removing chlorine from our water, because in their eyes the risk of contamination by microbes far outweighs the risks associated with cancer.

Pesticides, insecticides, herbicides and fungicides

The dioxins in herbicides promote testicular cancer. Among agricultural workers exposed to pesticides for twenty years or more, we find there is a significant risk they will contract cancers of the breast and pancreas. Those working in vineyards, however, are more likely to develop cancer of the bladder or brain, because different pesticides from those used in general agriculture are applied.

Cooking

The cooking process creates a shortage of micronutrients in our food by destroying a certain proportion of vitamins, and allows certain mineral salts and trace elements, particularly antioxidants that combat cancer, to leach away.

However, the cooking process also creates new substances in the food that could be suspect. Nowadays we are sure of the carcinogenic action on the intestines, of the benzopyrenes formed on meats, sausages or fish cooked on a grill or horizontal barbecue. In fact, anything that is grilled or toasted seems to be suspect - even toasted bread or coffee. The benzopyrene formed during the coffee roasting process could explain the high incidence of bladder cancers among heavy coffee drinkers.

Butter heated above 130°C produces acrolein, a carcinogen, and any cooking above 250°C will produce mutagenic substances that are responsible for cancers in the colon and rectum. If we want to minimise any carcinogenic risk, it is therefore advisable to cook at low temperatures, in a double boiler or steam.

When we cook foods containing a mixture of protein and carbohydrate (bread, for example), new substances are formed corresponding to the Maillard Reaction we get when we bake bread, which smell very good but could have a carcinogenic effect. However, the exact nature of this effect would depend on the amino acid and the carbohydrate involved.

Shortages of antioxidants

Any lack of antioxidants will make us vulnerable to cancer because without them we lack an important weapon in our fight against free radicals.

Nutrients that protect us against cancer

Fibre

Insoluble fibre (cellulose, hemicellulose) offers the most effective defence against cancer. The risk of contracting colonic-rectal cancer is reduced by 61% if the daily intake of fibre exceeds 20g.

Soluble fibre (like fruit pectin and the gum from dried vegetables) reduces the production of fatty acids that accelerate the growth of cancerous cells in intestinal cancers.

Antioxidants

It would appear that specific antioxidants help protect us from specific cancers, as indicated below:

ANTIOXIDANT	TYPE OF CANCER
Vitamin A	bladder, uterus
Vitamin C	lungs, larynx
Vitamin E	lungs, breast
Selenium	breast, uterus, lungs

Green vegetables

In addition to their antioxidants and fibre, green vegetables contain many other substances that protect us from cancer. Particularly noteworthy are:

• cabbage and broccoli

• cucumber

• parsley

• rosemary.

Fruit

Like green vegetables, fruit contains many substances, in addition to fibre and antioxidants, to help protect us from cancer.

To offer effective resistance to cancer

Eat wisely and avoid obesity.

Choose fish and meat, but neither smoked nor salted.

Reduce your intake of saturated fatty acids as much as possible.

Cut down intake of sugar and white flour as much as possible. Opt instead for carbohydrates with a low glycaemic index.

Enrich your diet with fibre (fruit, green vegetables, unrefined foods, pulses, organic bran).

Ensure a good intake of vitamins and micronutrients by eating as much raw food as possible, such as: crudités, fruit, salads, shellfish, fish (sushi) and meat (steak tartare).

Limit alcohol intake to two or three glasses of wine a day.

In conclusion, it is worth noting that this advice has much in common with a Mediterranean diet and is completely compatible with the general recommendations of the Montignac Method.

10 Avoid being undernourished

The nutritional balance of the body results from the balance between the chemical reactions of synthesis and degradation. Anabolism is the process of building up or repairing the cells of the body; catabolism is the process of wearing out or destroying those cells. Anabolism, particularly proteic anabolism, must be able to counterbalance catabolism and ensure the renewal of body structures. Undernourishment occurs just as much when anabolism diminishes as when catabolism increases in our body.

THE CAUSES OF UNDERNOURISHMENT

Inadequate intake (reduced anabolism)

Secondary anabolism of an intake of "vital substances" should normally keep protein mass stable and allow the building up of energy reserves for both the short and long term.

Anabolism can be reduced by inadequate nutritional intake brought about by:

- lack of appetite due to an infection, a depressive state or taking too much medication

- dietary choices that lead to the obsessive exclusion of certain foods

- bad teeth

- difficulty in swallowing

- poor digestive absorption (impairment of the small intestine, enzyme deficiency, spread of bacterial colic, difficulties in secreting insulin)

- emphysema, causing tiredness in the respiratory muscles

- a physical handicap that limits the ability to do the shopping, do the cooking, or even feed oneself

- socio-economic problems

- senility problems, affecting 20% of those over the age of eighty-five.

Accelerated use of protein stock (augmented catabolism)

This situation can be caused by:

• fever

• infection

• burns

• bedsores

• wounds that suppurate (leg ulcers, for example)

• fractures

• complications following an operation

• hyperactive thyroid

• inflammatory illnesses

• prolonged cortisone treatment

• cancer

• diabetes.

Any illness that becomes acute can suddenly change the metabolic balance of the body. Statistics show that of the elderly admitted to hospital to treat infections, 50% arrive undernourished and of those, 85% are hypercatabolic.

Moreover, as we have already seen, illnesses involve taking medication that can also give rise to further nutritional problems.

Which just shows how easy it is for an elderly person who falls ill, to pass rapidly from being well nourished to being worryingly undernourished. Added to which, the food you receive in hospital is not likely to reverse the process very much, as we see more cases of undernourishment in institutions than we do among those who are able to remain at home.

The consequences of being undernourished.

Undernourishment has important implications for health.

Immunodeficiency

This condition is due principally to a lack of protein, zinc, iron and vitamin B6. As a result, the reactions of the body to infection by a germ, virus or fungus are reduced owing to a reduction in the number of certain white corpuscles, to the level of interleukins 2 (substances secreted by certain white corpuscles, which stimulate their activity against infection) and to a reduction in the secretion of antibodies.

In the event of an infection, the body begins to secrete protein-consuming cytokinins that aggravate the process of hypercatabolism and destroy appetite, thereby adversely affecting anabolism by reducing food intake. We then find ourselves in a vicious circle, where the infection makes us even more undernourished and the risk of death is increased.

Healing

Undernourishment slows down the healing of wounds, ulcers, burns and surgical incisions.

Albumin synthesis

Albumin is a protein that makes medication more effective by transporting the active molecule. Lower levels of albumin in the blood will reduce the therapeutic effect of a medicine and increase its toxicity, which will be all the more difficult to eliminate because kidney function is often impaired with the elderly.

So what is the solution?

The best solution is obviously to prevent the elderly becoming undernourished, and this can be done by applying the following measures:

• provide a balanced diet, offering a wide variety of nutritious foods

• eliminate diets that are uninformed and too selective

- create material and psychological conditions that enable the patient to stay at home and be properly nourished

- take active steps to prevent infections (flu jabs)

- encourage the patient to develop an interest in nutrition and the pleasures of eating good food.

If undernourishment is diagnosed in time, is not severe and the patient does not have difficulty in swallowing, then the situation can be reversed fairly easily by ensuring the patient eats properly. If the patient has difficulties in swallowing, then a feeding tube may be necessary. In extreme cases, an intravenous drip may be the only solution.

Conclusion

The TGV from Paris to Marseille was rocketing down the track. It was early autumn, the clouds were low and the hills of Burgundy flew by, battered by torrential rain.

The young man opposite me stared fixedly out of the window. He seemed lost in his thoughts and his sad eyes suggested a certain melancholy in his soul.

To his left sat a woman you could not exactly call elderly, because it was so difficult to say how old she was. She talked continuously, gesticulating, joking and laughing at what she was saying to her husband facing her - a gentleman with a shock of silver hair, who found his wife so entertaining he never seemed to tire of her continual chatter. With a smile he nodded his head in agreement, occasionally contributing a brief comment, completing some detail, adding a point of his own. An unmistakable feeling of tenderness and happiness pervaded our compartment.

Suddenly the young man turned to them and said with great sincerity in his voice: "You are very lucky to be old!"

We all burst out laughing.

Appendices

Appendix 1
Have a nutritional check-up

When you read it, perhaps the chapter on the Montignac Method (page 109) seemed a trifle technical to you. However, you will now have realised that it contained indispensable information for a complete understanding of the nutritional needs of our body, particularly if our body has a certain inbuilt "maturity". Now that you have taken this on board, you will be able to take stock of your nutritional requirements so that you can put into operation the plan of campaign contained in Part 3 of this book.

Whenever the occasion arises, it is never too late to take our bearings; whether we are fifty, sixty or seventy years old, it is always wise to ask ourselves where we are and to pose the following questions:

• Am I, or am I not, in good health?

• What is the physical and intellectual state of my body?

• What do I eat?

DIETARY SELF-EXAMINATION

This can be the first stage of the check-up. When you have analysed your dietary habits or, better still, when you have gone through what you have eaten during the last couple of weeks with a fine-tooth comb, I suggest you identify:

Whether there is a certain harmony in your food selection

Whether you have any obvious dietary deficiencies

Whether there are any obvious excesses to correct.

The analysis of a traditional dietician using a software programme would give you a diet calculated to the nearest calorie as well as the proportion of each nutrient. However, together we will try to have a more general check-up, using the following questionnaire:

	Yes	No
Do you take 3 meals a day?	☐	☐
Do you have a large breakfast?	☐	☐
Do you eat cereals and/or bread at breakfast?	☐	☐
Do you eat a milk product (including cheese) 3 times a day?	☐	☐
Do you eat raw vegetables each day?	☐	☐
Do you eat a least 1 raw fruit each day?	☐	☐
Do you eat meat at least twice a week?	☐	☐
Do you eat fish at least twice a week?	☐	☐
Do you eat a cooked vegetable every day?	☐	☐
Do you eat a starchy food like rice, pasta, semolina or pulses, once a day either for lunch or dinner?	☐	☐
Do you eat unrefined foods (rice, pasta, bread)?	☐	☐
Do you use at least 2 different oils as dressing?	☐	☐
Do you use olive oil?	☐	☐
Do you use at least 10g of butter per day?	☐	☐
Do you limit your salt intake?	☐	☐
Do you limit your sugar intake?	☐	☐
Do you eat less than 3 lumps of sugar a day?	☐	☐
Do you drink 1.5 litres of liquid per day?	☐	☐
Do you drink 1-3 glasses of good wine per day?	☐	☐
Are you careful not to exceed 3 glasses (total 450cc) of beer or wine per day?	☐	☐
Do you refrain from drinking spirits such as gin, cognac and whisky?	☐	☐
Do you pay attention to the nutritional content of the foods you buy?	☐	☐
Do you ensure you buy organic foods?	☐	☐

Results:

Fewer than 6 affirmative answers:

It is high time you took a greater interest in your diet!

Fewer than 12 affirmative answers:

Your dietary habits are on the right track but you need to try harder!

More than 15 affirmative answers:

Very good. Just a little more effort and everything will be perfect!

More than 20 affirmative answers:

You are well on the way to reach a century.

YOUR PHYSICAL CONDITION

The expert eye of the "horse dealer" can be misled from time to time, as we saw earlier in the book, and corpulence should not lead us to make assumptions about how well nourished someone may, or may not, be.

What is so special about weight?

We have to be wary of our scales. It is, in fact, an inaccurate instrument as it only gives us an overall weight and does not tell us how much is fat, muscle or water.

Our weight can remain the same between the ages of twenty-four and thirty, whilst the composition of our body can change quite fundamentally. On average, the muscular mass of a man weighing 76 kilos can go from 24 to 13 kilos between the ages of thirty and eighty, and the fatty mass can change from 15 to 26 kilos during the same period. However, continuous sporting activity over the years can limit this loss of muscular mass.

As far as water is concerned, the amount in our bodies can vary a lot. It is low if the patient is dehydrated and high if the patient suffers from oedema.

Bone mass can also decrease by 2% - something that occurs with women suffering from osteoporosis.

This is why a thin person can have a well-fed body and an obese person can be undernourished. So we should never draw hasty conclusions from the fact that a person is overweight. Departments of the health service concerned with nutrition have a special piece of equipment called an impedometer to determine the proportion of body muscle, fat and water. The examination is quite simple: the patient lies down and is connected by electrodes to a machine that gives readings on different sectors of the body.

The Body Mass Index (or BMI)

This index is a way of assessing obesity by dividing weight in kilograms by height in metres squared (W/H^2). It gives a fairly accurate idea of the amount of fatty mass in the body.

A young male adult is considered to be:

Underweight   - with a BMI below 21

Slim   - with a BMI between 21 and 23

Normal   - with a BMI between 24 and 29

Obese   - with a BMI over 30.

The BMI of a young man weighing 70 kilos and 1.75m tall would be calculated as follows:

$W/H^2 = 70/3.06 = 22.8$

With a BMI between 21 and 23, this young man would be considered slim.

The BMI of a young man of the same height but weighing 90 kilos, would give us the following figure:

$W/H^2 = 90/3.06 = 29.41$

This indicates that he was on the verge of being obese.

Although this formula is helpful, it is still difficult to use over a certain age, as people, particularly women, have a tendency to shrink over the years. This loss of height is due to the compaction of the vertebrae caused by osteoporosis and women can lose up to 15cm in height. This is why, if we use the BMI as a way of measuring the elderly, we have to correct the factor height parameter, taking it back to the height recorded at the age of fifty.

A medical nutritionist or gerontologist could refine the data by measuring:

• cutaneous creases, indicating the thickness of the skin

• the surface area of the arm or the circumference of the calf, in order to assess muscle mass

• the minimum distance between heel and buttock when the knee is flexed.

Establishing the level of dehydration

Rough, dry skin, which makes the skin stay creased longer than normal when squeezed between forefinger and thumb, is indicative of dehydration. Conversely, some people may suffer from water retention, a condition that gives rise to swollen ankles.

More than 1.5 litres of urine should be produced over a period of twenty-four hours. A check should be made to ensure water intake is adequate.

Dental condition

Because they may lack teeth or have badly fitting false teeth, some people may have difficulty in chewing - an essential phase in the digestive process since:

• it increases the production of saliva, containing enzymes like amylase for example, which initiate the process of digesting starch

• it massages the gums and prevents teeth becoming loose

• it allows time for the flavour of food to pass into the nasal fossae, giving us a better chance to appreciate the aroma of foods and increase the pleasure of eating.

Now it is very important to preserve the hedonistic pleasure of eating. As Brillat-Savarin said: "The pleasures of the table belongs to every age, every condition, every country and every day: it can be linked with all the other pleasures and remains the last to console us when they are gone." Because our teeth are not quite up to the job, we should not then eat "soft" foods such as minced meat, mashes, soups and dairy products, which would reduce our need to chew.

Instead, we should pay a visit to the dentist to improve the state of our teeth as soon as possible. Someone with a depleted array of teeth and reduced chewing coefficient is very exposed to the dangers of malnutrition.

Laboratory tests

You make a point of ensuring your car has a periodic check-up to ensure it is functioning properly. Be keen to do the same for your body, because it deserves it.

Ask your doctor to prescribe a blood test to establish whether you are properly nourished or not. To do this, ask for the following checks.

- A blood count to uncover a possible anaemia caused by a lack of iron or vitamins B9 and B12, or perhaps a low level of white blood corpuscles.

- The level of iron in the blood, as well as ferritin, which increases iron reserves in the body.

- The level of folates, which could indicate a lack of vitamin B9.

- The ratio of creatinine in the urine with respect to height. If the ratio is too low, this would indicate a lack of protein.

- The level of albumin. If it is too low, this could be a sign that the patient is undernourished.

On the other hand, we can check for possible metabolic anomalies by measuring the:

- overall cholesterol level

- HDL cholesterol level

- triglyceride level

- blood sugar level

- insulin level

- uric acid level.

This way we will be able to detect diabetes, hyperlipidemia and the risk of gout or atheromata.

Other tests can be applied should your doctor think they are necessary, for example to determine sedimentation speed, which increases in the case of infection, inflammation or cancer, or to locate cancer tracers, particularly in the prostate.

X-Rays

An x-ray of the pelvis can show up stria characteristic of an osteomalacia caused by a lack of vitamin D. An X-ray of the pelvis or vertebrae can also show the existence of possible osteoporosis (most likely in the case of menopausal women not receiving hormone treatment).

However, the best way of assessing bone density and the severity of an osteoporotic condition or evaluate the risk of fracture (to the vertebrae and the neck of the femur) is to use a biphotonic absorption meter (a specialised scanner) that will also calculate body mass.

And lastly, X-rays make it easier to appreciate the severity of a degenerative osteoarthritis, which - if it is far advanced – might justify surgical intervention to replace a hip or knee.

Appendix 2
Understand the ageing process

How long can we expect to live?

In 1996, life expectancy for men was seventy-three and for women eighty-two. But, as we know, this statistic was an average which included all deaths regardless of how caused.

This means that if we exclude deaths caused by road accidents, which mainly involves those under the age of thirty, and particularly men, it is clear that the average age would go up quite substantially. This is why we can say with some certainty that a man of fifty can reasonably expect to live a further thirty years and a woman much more.

Terms such as "old" and "old age" often have a pejorative connotation. This is why they are often replaced by other words like "the elderly" or "the third age".

The expression "third age" was invented to describe that period of life when we go into retirement. It used to start at the age of sixty-five, set by law as the age at which men ended their active professional life, but as the age of retirement went down to sixty and then in some professional cases to fifty-five, this term has progressively lost its meaning.

But if we do not quite know where the third age begins, it is even more difficult to say where it ends. This is why some have even invented a "fourth age" to cover those quasi-mortals who thumb their noses at us by living beyond the age of eighty-five as they stride confidently towards three figures.

However, let us return to the original question: how long can we expect to live? If we compare ourselves to animals that have a life span five times the age at which they achieve physiological maturity, then we should be able to reach the age of a hundred and twenty without difficulty. And yet there are barely three thousand centenarians in France, where the incidence is one of the highest in the world. This is why the geriatrician could not resist letting slip when he examined some French patriarch or the other: "Could do better!"

Upon what does longevity depend? Two complementary hypotheses have been clearly put forward. That of Lamar, who maintains that our life expectancy is genetically programmed, and that of Darwin, who considers it to be dependent on our environment.

So, which part of the ageing mechanism is innate and which is acquired?

The factors involved in the ageing process

The genetic influence

To understand the life span of our cells, we must first of all study the phenomenon of their ageing process. In 1912, Alexis Carrel believed that cells could reproduce themselves indefinitely. But we had to wait until 1961 to share with Leonard Hayflick the certainty that our cells multiply by doubling no more than fifty times.

And to understand how these successive reproductions can give rise to a progressive change in our cells, all we had to do was look at the way a photocopier works. If we make successive photocopies of a text using not the original but the last copy we made, then the quality of the text will become progressively worse until eventually it becomes illegible. In this way, as our cells reproduce themselves, the original coded message changes and genetic mutations can appear. On the electron microscope, we can see the DNA containing our genetic codes breaking up in places and with each reproduction, the chromosomes lose small fragments called telomeres.

Admittedly, the body has at its disposal enzymes that can replace these losses. However, this maintenance system depends for its effectiveness on the immune system, which is normally in decline among the elderly, particularly if the quality of the food they are eating is poor.

However, although many cells such as skin cells, those of the mucous membrane and red blood corpuscles, are able to reproduce themselves, we must remember that brain, muscle and cardiac cells cannot do this: the same ones stay with us for the whole of our lives. Because they wear out of their own accord, we need to cosset them and protect them from being prematurely destroyed. Already from the age of twenty, we begin to lose neurones; from the age of twenty-four, we also begin to lose muscle cells.

Experiments involving the genetic modification of cells have allowed us to understand this phenomenon better. The mechanisms of cells wearing out and causing ageing are gene-dependent. However, we do not yet know whether this biological clock is controlled by an important number of genes or if one mutation of three genes, for example, is sufficient to trigger off the ageing process, like pulling the string on a detonator. A certain number of metabolic phenomena, more or less directly linked to food quality, could be behind genetically dependent cell degeneration.

In recent years, several experiments have been conducted, with mixed success, to try and arrest the ageing process.

1. Growth hormone

This hormone is secreted naturally by the body to stimulate the immune system, encourage the formation of scar tissue, consolidate bone and muscle structure and regulate fatty mass.

Secretion of our growth hormone declines with age. Volunteers who received three injections of this hormone a week over a period of six months saw their muscle mass increase by 10% and their fatty mass decrease by 14%. According to those around them, they appeared to have grown younger by ten to twenty years.

Unfortunately, the exorbitant cost of producing growth hormone makes it impossible for us to see how it can become universally available.

2. Melanin

This is the hormone that darkens the skin and is responsible for the pigmentation of the hair. White hair, usual after a certain age, indicates a deficiency in this hormone. An experiment showed that when mice in the laboratory were given melanin, their life span increased by 30%.

3. Dehydroepiandrosterone

Now, after fifty years, this substance is only manufactured at 30% of its original concentration. Injected into mice, it increased their lifespan by 20%. According to Professor Beaulieu, it will considerably reduce all signs of ageing in humans.

4. Stimulation of the immune system

When the immune system is undermined, our defences are weakened and we become more vulnerable to infections, because we have fewer T lymphocytes and are more receptive to cancer.

Ageing often results in us developing problems with our auto-immune system. In other words, our body starts to manufacture antibodies that begin to attack our organs uncontrollably.

The impact of the environment

When two identical cars come-off the production line, they do not have the same length of life ahead of them: everything depends on how they are driven, the kind of roads they follow, the climate conditions they endure and the quality of the maintenance they receive. They can be expected to cover 200,000 kilometres or perhaps only 80,000.

The potential lifespan written into our chromosomes may be a hundred and twenty, but when we are forty-five years old, our heart may already be worn out. So the lifespan of each one of us varies according to how well we have managed to look after ourselves.

There are several determining factors: pollution, stress, over-indulgence (tobacco addiction, alcoholism), but particularly bad dietary habits. Undernourishment can lead to poor immune defences and the production of free radicals, one of the main contributors to ageing.

Free radicals

There cannot be a single cosmetic promotion that does not mention free radicals. However, those that talk about them a lot do not necessarily seem to understand properly the role they play in the ageing process.

In the human body, electrons are organised into pairs, with one major exception: those associated with oxygen. In fact, oxygen is the only molecule that has unpaired, "celibate" electrons, called free radicals. Like all celibates, free radicals have but one idea: to find a mate. They therefore go off to "shack-up" with chromosome DNA and the lipids of cell membranes. The membrane lipids undergo a change. The walls of the cells oxidise and become more rigid, like rusting metal.

The outcome of all this aggression may be the death of the cell, which, as we know, is an objective cause of ageing. However, most of the time, the cell starts to function abnormally, providing an open door for many illnesses - blood pressure, arterial sclerosis, degenerative osteoarthritis and impaired cerebral function.

Fortunately our bodies can marshal a defensive strike force - a battalion of antioxidizing enzymes. But with age, the ranks of this battalion are thinned out and there are fewer and fewer antioxidizing enzymes ready to answer our call to arms.

Our diet could come to our aid by supplying antioxidants like betacarotene, vitamins C and E, selenium and zinc. Unfortunately, there is usually a lack of these micronutrients in modern foods, and particularly in the lifestyle too often adopted by the elderly.

Moreover, it is known that large numbers of free radicals are created as a result of:

• tobacco addiction

• alcohol addiction

• prolonged exposure to the sun (ultra-violet rays)

• naturally occurring ionising radiation

• pollution

• ozone.

We should also remember that immune deficiencies are encouraged by nutritionally poor diets, particularly those short in protein, iron and zinc. Which all goes to show how important our nutritional environment can be as we grow older.

For although our genes predispose, it is, in fact, our way of life that ultimately disposes.

Appendix 3
How to go shopping

As we have read this book, it has become increasingly clear that to avoid being undernourished we need to eat a very wide variety of foods. So, from now on, we must make a deliberate effort to see that we do precisely that.

The pleasure of eating

The exclusion of many foods from our diet as years go by - unless the process is based on sound medical grounds - can only end in shortages that will accelerate the ageing process or weaken our bodies and make them more vulnerable to disease.

Continued desire and pleasure are the best proofs that our passion for life remains unabated. It is why we must keep an open mind with regard to food and even a certain curiosity with regard to new foods. But to do this, we must guard against natural laziness that leads to monotony. We continue to make the same old dishes when we should make a point of fostering innovation by trying out some of the new recipes to be found in our magazines.

Here then, are a certain number of principles that, taken as a whole, should help us make an informed selection:

• Give a big place to raw foods: fruit, vegetables, oils (cold, first pressings) and even raw shellfish, like oysters. For cooking often involves structural changes that can change the nutritional quality of food (as with a carrot, for example), as well as cause a significant loss in nutrients.

• Consider restoring whole foods (cereals) as well as pulses, which are highly nutritious (lentils, haricot beans, split peas, chick peas)

• Rather than taking food supplements that are expensive and not always good for you, develop the habit of eating natural products on a daily basis - products that, as we have seen, have a high nutritional content, such as Brewer's yeast and wheatgerm.

Wise Shopping

In part two of our lives, we often have more free time on our hands. If this is so, we should use it profitably and wisely.

Above all, we must not forget our glasses, because we will need them to develop the habit of chasing labels, reading the wrappings - particularly the small print - and studying the list of ingredients: flour, sugar, starches, caramel, gums, additives, etc.

We should try to find out the nutritional content of the finished product. Are there any proteins? In what sort of quantities? Are the carbohydrates refined (white flour, sugar) or not? Are the lipids or fats saturated or polyunsaturated? What is the vitamin and mineral content? And what about trace elements?

The information you obtain may sometimes be surprising. It is doubtful whether you will continue buying packet soups - a nutritional catastrophe that should encourage you to go home and make your own. You will also discover vague notes, inaccuracies, not to speak of lies by omission, which have been perpetrated by manufacturers who prefer to suppress information that might discourage customers from buying their products.

By making a rigorous selection of products based on the guidelines given in this book, you will become an informed and responsible consumer rather than a "sucker" likely to be seduced by attractive yet misleading publicity.

The food industry has not yet come up with products specially adapted for those over fifty. However, it is not inconceivable that the situation may change for, with the "granny-boom" to come, the elderly will constitute a sizeable market - a market that will be all the more coveted because this social category will have a not inconsiderable disposable income with food high on its agenda. Furthermore, if the birth rate continues to stay low in the years to come (1.6 babies per woman), in fifty years, those over sixty will represent a third of the population.

When shopping for food today, we often have a wide choice of outlets to choose from.

The small shopkeeper

The small shopkeeper has the great advantage of being close at hand, something that is very important for those with mobility problems, and they continue to provide important services such as delivering heavy items to your door. The small shopkeeper also has the chance to exchange the time of day with customers, something that can help break the heavy loneliness that afflicts quite a few people.

The local market

For those lucky enough to have one, the local market is still the most magical place to do your shopping: a symphony of colours, varied smells, wide choice and animated conversation. Before buying, you can go right round the market to see what is on offer, comparing quality and prices. We can also choose to go to the local farm shop (which may sell organic produce) where the food should be very fresh and nutritious, coming - as we are led to believe - from the immediate locality.

The supermarket

The supermarket may have the advantage of being cheaper and offering a wider variety of products. However, the down side is you need a car to get there and it is not always easy to find your way around. Furthermore, qualitative choices are not always easy to make, as prices cannot be compared. However, it is the ideal place to scrutinise labels carefully.

The over-sixty-year-olds tend to be fairly traditional in culinary matters, but should not be completely suspicious when confronted by progress. Here again, we need to take everything into account. All suspicions regarding chemical preservatives are reasonable, but similar reservations regarding deep frozen foods are completely exaggerated. Produce frozen a few hours after picking, is often richer in vitamins than a fresh product harvested before it ripe to help it cope with several days' transport.

Take time, shop with care and be demanding about the quality and nutritional content of the food you buy. In doing so, you will help form wholesale distribution and, indirectly, the food industry.

Do not choose a food simply because it is easy to prepare or so-called "oven-ready". There is a great difference between eating and knowing how to feed yourself. Brillat-Savarin used to say: "The animal feeds, man eats, but only a wise man knows how to eat." Let us guard and keep up that philosophy, by preparing meals with an Epicurean dimension. Let us eat with knowledge and discernment, if possible in a convivial environment, guarantor of a healthy appetite and the joy of sharing.

Life in an institution

So far in this book, we have scarcely touched on the problem of people who have no choice regarding the food they eat. They are those that have council meals delivered to their home, or eat in community day centres, nursing homes or other institutions for the elderly.

These people are unfortunately not responsible for putting their meals together and therefore have to eat what they are given. If they feel the composition of their meals is unsatisfactory, apart from organising a strike or revolt, it should always prove possible for them to balance their diet according to our recommendations, by making adjustments either at breakfast time or with a snack between meals.

When we are aware of the problem and are able to buy additional food either directly or indirectly, a solution is always possible providing we have the will to improve our diet.

Appendix 4
The protein and fibre content of food

AMOUNT OF PROTEIN IN 100G OF FOOD

Animal protein		Vegetable protein	
Horse	20g	Soya seed	35g
Beef	20g	Wheatgerm	25g
Veal	20g	Oats	13g
Pork	17g	Germinated rye	13g
Lamb	15g	Germinated wheat	12g
Cooked ham	18g	Germinated barley	10g
Raw ham	15g	Corn on the cob	9g
Black pudding	24g	Wholemeal bread	9g
Saucisson	25g	Wholemeal pasta	8g
Chicken	20g	Haricot beans	8g
Egg	6g	Lentils	8g
Fish	20g	Chick peas	8g
Dutch cheese	35g	Kidney beans	8g
Gruyere	35g	White bread	7g
Brie	20g	Semolina	5g
Camembert	20g	White pasta	3g
White cheese	9g	Whole rice	7g
Yoghurt	5g	White rice	6g
Milk	3.5g	Muesli	9g
Petits-Suisse	9g	Tofu	13g
Mussels	20g	Soya flour	45g
Shrimps	25g	Soya milk	4g
		Soya germ	4g

We should eat 1 gram of protein for every kilo of our body weight, per day, with lower and upper limits set at 60g and 90g respectively. Thus a woman weighing 50 kilos should eat 60g per day; a woman of 65 kilos, 65g per day; a man of 80 kilos, 80g per day; a man of 110 kilos, 90g per day.

FIBRE CONCENTRATION IN SOME PRINCIPLE FOODS

Cereal products		Pulses		Dried and oily fruit	
Bran	44	Raw dried beans	25	Dried apricots	24
Unrefined cereals	11	Cooked dried beans	4.5	Dried coconut	23
Unrefined flour	9.5	Raw split peas	23	Dried figs	18.3
Oats	7.2	Raw chick peas	22	Prunes	16
Wholemeal bread	6.5	Cooked chick peas	6	Almonds	14
Tinned maize seed	5.7	Dried lentils	12	Hazelnuts	9
Brown bread	5	Cooked lentils	4	Dates	8.7
Whole rice	4.5	Cooked kidney beans	3.5	Black olives	8.2
Corn flakes	3			Peanuts	7.5
White bread	2.7			Raisins	6.8
White rice	2			Walnuts	5
				Green olives	4.4

FIBRE CONCENTRATION IN SOME PRINCIPLE FOODS

Fresh fruit		Vegetables and Tubers	
Coconut	13	Celery	6
Raspberries	7.4	Garden peas	5.3
Gooseberries	6.8	Cooked spinach	5
Pears with skin	3	Cabbage	5
Oranges	2.9	Broccoli	4.3
Apples	2.5	Lamb's lettuce	4.3
Peaches	2.3	Artichoke	4.2
Bananas	2	Raw potatoes	3.5
Other fruit	< 2	Cooked potatoes	1
		Carrots	3.4
		French beans	7.2
		Leeks	3.1
		Other vegetables	< 3

Index

abdomen 22

abdominal pain 44

aches 25

acidifying foods 75-6

acidosis 75, 85

acids 21, 33

additives 9

adolescence 17, 119, 151, 153

adrenal glands 39

aggressiveness 69

alcohol 26, 29, 30, 32, 48, 53, 56, 57,
58, 61, 75, 76, 77, 124, 128, 129,
137, 149, 155, 159, 186, 187-8,
191, 211, 212

algae (seaweed) 33, 43

alimentary
process 20
tract 23

alkalising foods 75-6

allergies 25, 71

almond oil 40

almonds 42, 45, 51, 52, 61, 62, 64,
75, 79, 98, 134, 135, 136, 149,
218

alphalinoleic acid 42

aluminium 95, 97

Alzheimer,s disease 50, 72, 97

amino acid 189

anaemia 96

anorexia 21, 25, 69

antibiotics 9, 25, 58, 75, 178

anti-coagulants 25

anti-depressants 53

antihistamines 71

antioxidants 26, 50, 51, 52, 73, 95,
130, 134-5, 137, 140, 149, 165,
181, 187, 188, 189, 190, 212
menu 134-5

anxiety 37, 69, 70, 71, 107

aphrodisiacs 89-94

appetite 21, 27, 37, 57, 96, 192

apples 51, 133

apricots 45, 51, 52, 62, 64, 77, 134,
135, 218

arterial
hypertension 70
lesions 42, 137

arteries 36, 40, 126

arthritis 20, 24

artichokes 62

asparagus 75

aspirin 63, 75, 137, 167

asthma 71

atheroma 126, 130, 147, 157

auto-immune illnesses 177

avocados 79

baby-boom generation 8, 12, 14, 18

bananas 62, 115

barbecues 182

barley 35, 43

Books written by Michel Montignac and translated into English, which are now on sale in the United Kingdom.

Dine Out and Lose Weight
ISBN 290623634-9   224pp -RRP £12.95

Michel's first book, originally released in France in 1986 and intended for the busy executive with an active weight problem. The English version has been revised recently, to make it more comprehensive and easier to read. For medics and nutritionists, there is an extended technical appendix at the end. A quality production, attractively presented, it remains a particularly suitable gift for the busy professional.

Eat Yourself Slim... and Stay Slim!
ISBN 291273700-1   240pp - £12.00

This new title builds on the success of *Eat Yourself Slim* (first published in 1989) and brings the Montignac method completely up to date.

The core message remains the same, but much new material has been added. Tables have been extended and greater attention has been given to the long term application of the Method - hence the amended title. In addition, readers are also introduced to a new concept called the Average Glycaemic Index, which replaces the 'discrepancy management' of earlier books. This new concept is intended to help those embarking on Phase II widen their selection of food without straying too far beyond the bounds of good Montignac dietary practice.

Published in September 1998, *Eat Yourself Slim...and Stay Slim!* has become very popular with established and new Montignac followers alike, showing itself a worthy successor to the title it replaces.

The Montignac Method - *Just for Woman*
ISBN 291090700-7   328pp - £11.95

This book was first published in France in 1994 and was written by Michel, to address the difficulties sometimes experienced by women with a more delicately balanced hormonal system. In addition to the help it gives women to return permanently to normal weight, it is also a goldmine of advice on how to keep young and healthy through a wise choice of foods.

It is the first book in which Michel begins to apply his pioneering dietary work to the broader field of overall health. Published in English in 1995, this book has recently moved into second position on the Montignac 'best-sellers' list.

The Miracle of Wine
ISBN 290623664-0   256pp - RRP £15.00

The title of this book is drawn from a chapter in his first book *Dine Out and Lose Weight*, dealing with the health-giving properties of wine. Michel returns to a topic that still continues to fascinate. Written primarily for a French audience, its appeal and relevance are universal.

With 12 pages of colour, it is the ideal coffee-table book to compliment *Dine Out and Lose Weight*.

Recipes & Menus
ISBN 290623662-4   285pp RRP - £15.00

Still very popular, this is Michel's first cookbook, written to support those following the method. As its title suggests, there is an extended eating plan incorporating the recipes in the book. Illustrated in colour.

Montignac Provençal Cookbook
ISBN 290623684-5   336pp - £25.00

This hardback, all-colour cookbook, underlines Michel's gastronomic credentials. Designed to compete head-on with the best mainline cookery books, it has the advantage of being entirely compatible with the dietary method and includes a three-month eating plan. Particular care has been given to ensure recipes are not only clear and concise, but also quick and easy to produce. A classic.

The above titles can be obtained from all good bookshops. In the event of difficulties, please contact our UK distributors

JH Haynes & Co Sparkford
Order line: Telephone 01963 442105
Facsimile 01963 440001
sales@haynes-manuals.co.uk

VISIT

The Montignac Boutique & Café
Gourmet food store, Café & Wine Bar

160 Old Brompton Road
London SW5 0BA

Telephone/Fax 020 7370 2010
www.montignac.co.uk
mail@montignac.co.uk

For

Montignac wine and provisions, including bread.
Hot and cold drinks, snacks and meals all day.
Hot and cold food to take away.

A la Carte dining in the Wine Bar
Mondays to Saturdays – evenings only.

Store opening Hours
Mondays - Fridays 8.30-9.00pm
Saturdays 8.30 - 6.00pm
Sundays 10.00 - 5.00pm

Mail Order
Via the above website, or call for catalogue.

*Everything available in the boutique is
compatible with the Montignac Method.*